T0116162

The Diamond Path

A Guide to the Art of Healing

First Edition

Magnolia May Polley

Order this book online at www.trafford.com
or email orders@trafford.com

Most Trafford titles are also available at major online book retailers.

Print information available on the last page.

ISBN: 978-1-4120-8188-7 (sc)

Trafford rev. 04/17/2019

Trafford PUBLISHING® www.trafford.com

North America & international
toll-free: 1 888 232 4444 (USA & Canada)
fax: 812 355 4082

I dedicate this book to all of those who continue to dream and to my family who have always encouraged me.

❧

When the trail gets long,
Remember why you travel.
When your hands are wet with sweat and tears,
Remember why you toil.
On the day you wake without fear,
Remember who you are.
On the day the stars shine for you,
Remember the rhythm.

Table of Contents

Prelude

A grand circle exists between all of those who are taking part in life at this time. We are the fortunate ones. We are the chosen ones. It has taken a long time for me to put my arms around that simple truth. So many organisms, molecules, and elemental mechanisms never have a chance at much more than reaction. A human being has the most opportunity to experience life in a fulfilling, cognitive, intentional, and free way. We do have social boundaries and laws that exist through out all cultures that seem unjust and rigid; forces that seem to shape our lives and control our existence. We must teach ourselves how to become master navigators, manifestoes, and investors in our own fate. The more we blame others for their influence or control over our lives the more we create situations that are never handled. It is easier to pass the blame and hold grudges than it is to take real responsibility. We must take control of our lives on our own terms. We must rediscover the magic and fascination that is a part of the beautiful universe we live in. We must find what makes us joyous. We must take responsibility for the actions that keep us alive and enjoying. We must do our life's work and know that the world is better for it afterwards.

The Earth is an amazing guide. The Earth is a burial site of tools, stories, and ideas that are all a piece of the puzzle. These pieces are constantly shifting and being reset by new hands with different ways of looking at things. I am just one set of eyes and hands. I have been watching, listening, and searching for my own truth. I have moved forward and I have moved backwards, but I have always stood firm in the belief that I am a part of something astonishing that deserves exploration. This is the beauty of life on Earth.

I am continually fascinated by what the world is teaching me and I hope to get the sparks of imagination flying by offering a collection of traditional ideas rearranged in a way that speaks a new truth. I look at the space around me as a great mystery becoming more and more familiar, filled with uncountable treasure chests of beauty and knowledge that are just waiting to be opened.

Scope and Focus

I am dedicated to doing my part in helping to make the healing arts receivable and usable by everyone. In this book, I include the basic science behind color, light, and the circadian rhythms. I will also talk about the art of working with the body's aura, the pendulum, diamonds as healers, jewelry as medicine, and prayer and manifestation. This grouping of work will also include poems and personal stories that I hope will be encouraging to the reader.

I have always believed that I have a livelihood as a body worker because families and communities do not have the time or space to develop ways to take care of themselves effectively or efficiently. I encourage people to stop at no ends to create health and balance in the lives of themselves and those they care for.

My hope is that people who practice within the field of healing, as well as people interested in keeping up with their own health will see some truth in what is laid out in the pages that follow. This is also a book that will encourage those sitting on mounds of treasure or old boxes of family jewelry to sift through and find meaning in what they wear and keep. My way has never been the only way, but it is a way that can make the mystery of healing understandable to those who discount it or who think that the information they have read in the past holds too little substance. This is the kind of reading that will stick to your spiritual ribs and will nourish the soul and mind for many days to come!

My queries with the "unknown" have kept me up many a night; and made me curse traditional medicine and religions of all kinds. I have lost faith in myself and all others—questioned their true motives and my own many times, just to come full circle each time with one great and simple truth. Although there are some universal truths, most things are individual truths. Everything we learn must be sorted and organized to fit our own circuitry, literally. Some information is right for us and some is more difficult to understand. This does not mean that any concept should be completely abandoned. Everything has a purpose and a time.

I am no expert. I do know what helps me to climb the mountains of endless questions and answers. I know what makes sense to me when the rest falls away. I follow a genuine path---I try always to be honest with myself if nothing else. The fundamentals in this book are those that work well for me. This is the way I understand and live in the world around me. My hope is that I can provide clarification to readers who have a limited base of understanding in the ways of healing. I respect the teachings I have, but I know that there is much to learn. I am learning and I am teaching, I know that this will always be true. I am a single human who wants to encourage others to consider alternative medicine and healing. This is an art form, a science, a myth and a mystery wrapped into one. I hope that you can appreciate these universal truths. I look to offend no one and my expression is for the good of all. May light shine upon every individual path of discovery.

An Introduction: Bodywork

Before a person can be a facilitator of healing, they must have a general understanding of anatomy and physiology. This not only makes the individual credible, but more accurate when focus and intention are required. One does not need to become a doctor, physical therapist or massage therapist to accomplish this goal. Home study and taking anatomy and physiology classes at a local college can be sufficient for gathering this type of knowledge.

My first love will always be bodywork. So much is improved by circulation. All of the tissues that make up our bodies are crying out for more oxygen and more water. Life begins with our first breath and ends with our last breath; this breath carries with it the pure essence of life. Receiving massage is like allowing your body to take a full deep breath of life. Exercise of any kind is an ideal, but many of us cannot make the time to stretch, exercise, vacation, or even rest. Massage is an organized time for renewal and relaxation. Most of us are not able to schedule our days full of balancing activities like yoga, tai chi, meditation, massage, or even a morning tea. We need to choose to do what we can. Our society has built a structure of people who do not have time to stop, and if they do, it is for a drink or a cigarette. It is not that taking time for guilty pleasure is necessarily bad, it is that no one feels guilty about a drink or a smoke; they feel guilty about taking time to care for themselves. This is a backwards way of thinking and it is becoming the norm. If we want to have a drink without consequence to our bodies, we have to take care of ourselves during the meantime, so that we have the stamina to process the garbage out of our bodies. If there is more garbage than healthy substances in our bodies, our human bodies become more like garbage. We become lumps of uselessness. If we don't put in enough nutrients, our bodies are naturally in a state of starvation for energy and will try to turn the coffee, alcohol, processed foods, and smoke covered material into something usable, breaking us down over time. We cannot afford to take these things into the cellular structure of our bodies. Massage and other alternative healing techniques can help many individuals to process this kind of waste out of the body more quickly.

Massage allows the blood to move freely, rehydrating and providing oxygen to needy cells. Ligaments, tendons, cartilage, muscles, and the skin are gifted with the freedom of movement, allowing the individual to experience a heightened state of health. Western medicine and natural medicine, including massage, are not on the same page. Your body needs oxygen and water to repair itself and to clean itself. Synthesized pharmaceuticals and surgery can actually complicate the body's natural mechanism of survival by creating major roadblocks in the form of real trauma rather than repair. Surgery and heavy duty pharmaceuticals should be a last resort after all else has failed, but instead they are primary methods of care. The field that I work in, repairs the people who come stumbling, damaged, and angry by the out and out abuse put on them by traditional western medicine. This is no joke; I have no choice but to be reminded every day by my clients on how barbaric and crude western medicine can be. What happened to the wise old doctor who took care of generations of family members? These keepers of patterns, remedies, and family trees seem to have disappeared like the Pueblo Indians. Corporations full of greed and empty promises have replaced these Kind and giving souls. It doesn't sound good, does it? I am begging MD's to give the disappointed a reason to sing a more chipper tune and cheer. I feel like I am riding a big lazy wave into shore, right on the brink and looking towards a land of New Hope. I am no doctor. I am a caregiver, working on the side of progression for humanity and I encourage everyone interested in or a part of western medicine to open their eyes to the true wisdom of common sense. If your family practitioner is golden, then you have a real treasure, hold on to the people who are searching for the answers that aid the individual, rather than the ones that hope to saturate the public with unknown formulas of potential poison. I have met doctors who are progressive and do embrace the alternatives. My hope is that one day these hybrid doctors will replace the ones who most of us seek today for general care.

Many people are receiving massage and other alternative therapies because they are happy with the positive results they experience. Pain and stress are two things that can be managed with great success through bodywork. If we could let go of some of our pain and stress, life would be more enjoyable. Pain and stress cause most of our sick days and many of our arguments. When we feel taken care of, we are more likely to give to others. I look foreword to putting smiles on the faces of my clients, sending them out with a better over-all feeling that lasts the whole day and usually much longer. Getting into the habit of giving back to ourselves makes it possible for us to feel like there is room to give to someone else and to be happier by doing it. When we feel less pain and stress we smile and laugh more; we hold the door open for someone else to pass; we treat our families and friends better, and we are more productive during work. The ultimate payback for a massage therapist is hearing that your clients are going home and massaging their children and their mates. I am happy to be a part of a real movement of positive action that is working its way forward.

One

A History of Healing

There have always been groups of people who live together. Usually, the caretaker or healer will rise within a group when there is a need for them. If a baby is sick or an old woman is unable to walk, the healer or caretaker will always do what they can to help the unfortunate to survive. This is the natural empathetic nature of the healer. Pushed by their personal conviction and character the healer takes interest in foods and exercises that promote wellness and eventually will form remedies for illness and pain. Some societies have shunned these people; some have put them on pedestals. Perhaps, it has always been about how the healer of the group develops his or her skill and their individual ability to apply it that has dictated the survival of the tribe.

"Sacred plants are often a vital ingredient in shamanic healing rituals and so are magical helper spirits or allies," says Neville Drury. If a practice became something of an oddity or a death occurred the group would accuse the healer of ill intentions or foul play would soon be suspected throughout the group. If a remedy worked, the healer would receive social honor and reverence. "Indian doctors were honored by their group by having give-aways or pot-lucks. Families would bring their best foods or sacred gifts in honor of the Indian doctor or shaman. Many tribes of the Pacific Northwest pass medicine through family lineage; from grandfather to son and so on," exclaims Beaver Chief, a traditional Indian doctor.

I would like to re-tell a well-known story of the ancient healing practice of Shiatsu that has roots in Japan. Originally, bodywork was reserved for the blind men of Japan. Armed with a whistle and their hands, these body specialists would stand on street corners and toot until someone would come to them interested in their service. This has been a custom for thousands of years and the story was originally passed down to me during a Shiatsu class. The blind were favored because they have no judgment of beauty or disability; their sight seems to go much deeper than this. The distractions of physical attribute are removed and what is left are the hands and intuition of the healer and the body of the client. Trying to imagine a world of people without eyes can seem unfortunate, but we as the human race would be forced to let go of prejudices and focus much more on the feelings we receive and send out. What would be left in our interaction with others, but sound and touch? We would have to form our worlds cognitively around touch, smell, taste, and sound.

I personally know that I can do some of my best work completely in the dark or with my eyes closed. It is lovely to watch a body worker move and massage with pure intention and confidence with their eyes shut. This is a beautiful kind of dance. Once a body worker performs this sacred dance with passion and intention towards the true well being of another, few things can replace their feelings of gratitude and wholeness. Who are these body workers and medicine people who have lived for centuries within each tribe and civilization? These are the people who love humanity, who look to make improvements within our social structures, who know that by showing true love and understanding towards the folks they encounter will only bring about more love and understanding.

> *May we all look at one another through eyes without fear and*
> *judgment.*
> *May we touch other people with knowledge so ancient, it has no*
> *source.*
> *May we always be in touch with ourselves enough to see that we*
> *deserve as much as the next person.*
> *May we all be encouraged to take care of our selves, our families, our*
> *communities, and our planet.*
> *May the search for knowledge go on.*
> *May we find joy everyday in something.*
> *May those who heal be celebrated.*

Two

Stones: Harnessing Earth Energy

"The dreams of magic may one day be the waking realities of science"

SIR JAMES FRAZIER

It was during my studies of anthropology that I began to see patterns in the use of burial mounds, stone circles, sacred circles, pyramids, etc. These are all sacred places and were all built with different intentions in mind, mostly protection and as energy modulators. Many cultures incorporate sacred geometry and mathematics into the construction of their mounds, circles, and structures. There was a time when nothing was done without the expression of intention and everything was ceremonial and sacred. Stones have been used to communicate with the heavens, other humans, and to create manifestation on the earthly planes. A stone holds a vibration that keeps rhythm with the earth. Half-exposed and half-buried—the stone presents a unique opportunity for humans to experience the Earth's energy. Stones act as memorials and blessings. They can also be landmarks for people so that they never forget an event or an important place. Land markers made of stone are known as cairns. America's most current use of standing stones is within our national parks as trail markers and in our cemeteries to honor our deceased.

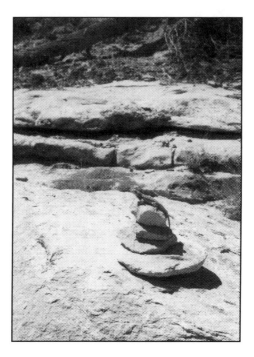

A cairn or trail marker in Canyonlands, Utah

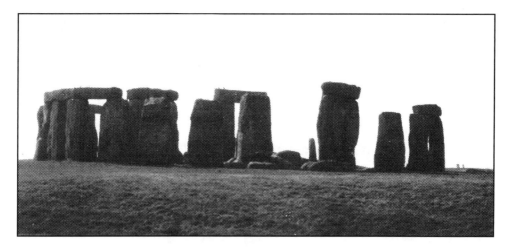

Stonehenge at dawn Wessex, England

The standing stone circles in the world draw visitors from all backgrounds of interest. We all have our speculations as to exactly what these circles significance are. I agree with the idea that these stones are time-stones, meant to give signal to the rising and setting of the mid-winter and mid-summer sun, as well as all kinds of astronomical phenomenon. The people brought these large stones to places on the Earth that were sacred and the energy was harnessed for reasons such as protection and healing, possibly departure/death as well. The circles being made of stone are very high in Quartz crystal making the theory of energy conduction in Atlantis plausible. I hold the belief that if one puts a large stone made of Quartz half in the ground and half out of it and one places many of these stones in a circle over a place known to have connecting ley lines and under-ground water sources, you have created an energy generator. Leys or ley lines are straight lines of energy that are found within the Earth and emit an electro-magnetic frequency that can be picked up by a dowsing tool, such as an angle wire or willow branch. People today use these tools to find underground water sources, as well. My family has relied on water-witchers, or people who can use a dowsing tool, to find underground water sources for the drilling of wells on our property in Washington State for decades.

Stones that have inclusions of crystals oscillate due to the natural ebb, pull, and flow of the magnetics that are continually moving from North to South within our Earth. This keeps our Earth spinning and perfectly round in its orbit, transferring the pulsing energy of the magnetics within the Earth to these stones, which have been used forever to hold various vibrations, such as those at Stonehenge. It is only natural to believe that these oscillators are being used as a great timekeeper, much like the quartz clocks or a driving force for something that needed regulation through pure energy. Geometrical shapes have been found all over the world and with precision each of them were built to generate energy. Earth Energy. The Earth spins due to the magnetics that exist within it, why is it a stretch to see that this energy cannot only affect you and I, it can be harnessed and used by the those that seek to understand it. Consider how much effort the U.S. puts into making sure we have the energy to keep our society moving and capable of sustaining our culture. This is not a new idea and I plan to encourage each student that searches for understanding to walk away with the tools they need to heal themselves and one another using what is spinning right under our feet. Once we learn to harness this naturally renewing energy source, we can learn to heal our communities, the world, and ourselves. Humans were not so distracted at one time; there were many more of us who dedicated their lives to the great mysteries of the Earth. Circles are universally used to mark a sacred space. Sacred structures are built to last the ages so that no one will forget their power. Our responsibility is to identify these places and spend time figuring out the spiritual side of these monuments. Passion and spirit drives everything, even an excessive use of resources, like the great pyramids.

We all should know about the great intensity of the pi symbol. Pi is the result of any equation that passes into infinity and has a place in many great mysteries. Magnificent studies have been done on the pyramids that prove it was not just the people of Egypt that were amazing; the structures themselves were geometrically amazing, as well. William Wilks, a man who spent his retirement focusing on geomancy, magnetics, and dowsing, found that it is the shape of the pyramid itself that creates energy. However, this energy was not found to be positive for healing or for life in general. Acting as a dehydration tool a pyramid can somehow diffuse the oxygen in the air within it causing an absence of decay in any way to what ever is left inside of it. Wilks found this to be an energy that promotes mummification through a change in the cellular movement. This created a slowing of degeneration, like a natural dehydrator for inanimate objects, such as vegetables. This only happened during his experiments when he placed the triangular structure in a position of true north to south alignment. I encourage those interested in this subject to read his book, *The Science of a Witches Brew.*

I mentioned previously that underground water is one of the elements that people find at sacred sights with a dowsing tool. Alfred Watkins has found a different kind of energy associated with the lines in the earth called leys. Watkins has published a fabulous book on the subject called, *The Old Straight Track.* Many researchers who study sacred sites have found that energy is associated with these lines. Leys of energy are six to eight feet wide and are considered to have yang energy while underground water lines were considered yin. Many times the two types of lines are found together. It is where veins of water cross with energy leys that create the energy of a sacred sight. These conditions are found at sacred sights reaching as far apart as Machu Picchu, the circular underground kivas of the Anasazi, the stone circles of Britain, the high alter of Charte cathedral in France and the stone labyrinths of Sweden. Dowsers all read individually just like an individual practicing divination through tarot, runes, etc. (Dowsing the Way, By: Sig Lonegren).

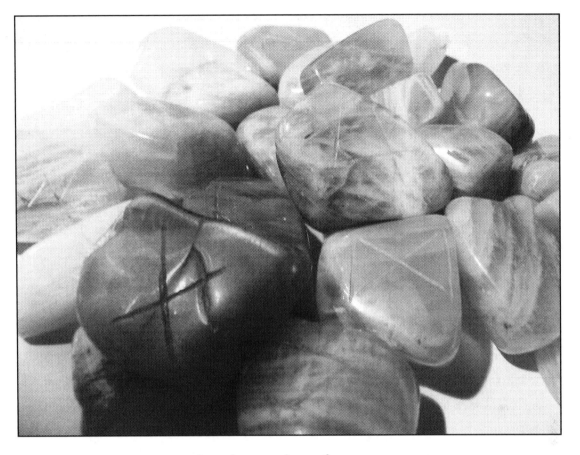

A set of runes made out of moonstone

The Mekigar or men of magic live in the Northern areas of Australia and they hold the quartz crystal in high regard as "wild stones" and forms of solidified light. These medicine men use quartz, australite, and stones and bones as power bearers known to hold rich symbolic significance. Quartz is thought to embody the Great Spirit. The Mekigar's education consists of sorcery and diagnostic techniques in the cure of illness and psychic disorder. These are the important social contributions that the Mekigar gives to his community in the role of doctor (*The World Atlas of Divination*, by: J. Matthews).

At Wookey Hole Caves in Somerset, England, recent archaeological excavations revealed a woman's skeleton dating back to the Stone Age. With her bones was an artificially polished sphere of crystalline granite about the size of a baseball (*Wise Women Counselors*, Marion Green). We can assume that this was used as a magical charm and tool for divination.

Dhyani Ywahoo, a woman who represents the Cherokee teachings, writes in her book,

Voices of our Ancestors, "The crystal works on the parasympathetic nervous system through the optic nerve. The eyes absorb the light energy beyond the visible light spectrum. The peripheral vision is more sensitive to the subtle energy of life, such as auras, energy is absorbed through the peripheral vision, and even if the child is born blind or traumatized, the subtle body still has those functions. The peripheral vision's reception of light directly affects the pineal and pituitary glands. We can visualize a little cup within the mind, which is receiving subtle energy and distributing it through the entire endocrine system. Human beings like crystals are energy generators. Just as the crystal emits negative ions that carry away the unhealthy charge around the environment, so can we, through clarifying our own thought and our nature. The crystals polarization, the way it receives the light, determine how the spirals energy meet around particular planes and call from within the wholeness of white light the colors needed by the individual." The Ywahoo believe that only people who are mentally and spiritually clear should be trusted with the use of crystals for healing, mainly their own people.

The Earth has provided us with many tools for healing. In fact, the whole of the Earth is a composite of elements that can be used and harnessed for energy. It is possible to teach ourselves non-destructive ways to use the energy spinning under our feet to heal all of the organisms that depend upon our Earth and to gain a greater understanding of the nature of the elements and the energy they create and emit. The possibilities are endless and can be reflected in the great stone circles, pyramids, Mayan and Inca temples, under ground water sources and ley lines, fault lines, and volcanoes. We already collect energy from the movement of water and wind. We can use sunlight to charge our solar panels. One day, we may be able to replace fossil fuels with energy that we collect from earthquakes and lightening.

Three

Basic Principles of Energy and Wavelengths

Light is energy. We know that light is a visible electro-magnetic wave. A long wavelength on the lowest frequency visible is called infrared light. Ultra-violet light, on the other hand, vibrates on the highest frequency and produces the shortest wavelength. All other light falls between ultra-violet and infra-red. Light polarizes all molecules that it encounters, a process that slows down its speed.

When someone is observing or using a gemstone for healing, the light they see naturally flowing through the gemstone slows down significantly due to its index of refraction. Refraction creates color. A diamond's index of refraction or ability to reflect light is one of the elements used to decipher its worth. Transparent materials tend to polarize more easily. As the light enters a crystal, it begins to refract creating a spectrum of color and deferring the light from traveling in the straight line of its original destiny. This reaction creates a miniature field of its own, offering us harnessed energy to utilize. Therefore, by harnessing polarized sunlight energy from a controlled light substance, one is able to create a unit of dispersible energy. Light is recognized by its color. Color is produced by how quickly or slowly the light is moving. This is called the frequency. Visible light is found between 400-800 nanometers or 250-2400 Hertz. The Hertz vibration determines color and all living organisms emit vibrations at a frequency between 300-2000 nanometers. Scientists call this energy the biofield. Body workers call this field the aura. White light is a representation of all the colors and when one shines this light through a faceted crystal, with each inclusion or barrier the light wave hits, the light is slowed and broken down, creating an array of colors all vibrating at different frequencies. These are the colors or the subtle energies that body and energy workers are attempting to work with. Every living organism creates an amount of light that is emitted from within and depends upon the complexity of its molecular structure. So, just as the Sun sends us a life-giving amount of polarizing energy, our bodies naturally emit a small amount of that energy on its own.

According to Colour Energy Corporations, a company that produces alternative UV light sources such as bulbs and light pens, "In a positive sense the organs are supplied with the missing bio-energy that is needed for proper functioning. The organs can be contacted and mended by using the color wand with crystal lenses to focus the color energy to the corresponding chakra. This procedure washes each energy center out with clean, charged, polarized, pure colored light. Thus, affecting our bodies in a positive way by contacting its molecular mechanisms through simple vibration."

What can be more harmless than this? It seems that the process of refraction acts like a filter for the raw intense light, breaking it down into frequencies that our bodies can use and handle. This is why light is an effective tool that we can use to promote health within any living organism and why the healing community has used it traditionally for centuries.

Four

The Importance of Light and Healing

An old Inuit tale tells of the malnutrition and severe depression that comes from the long lightless winters in Alaska and Northern Canada. An over-sized flesh-eating monster, Wendigo would come when the people were hungry and desperate in the middle of winter and it would make the people into crazy cannibals who fed on the flesh of the dying. Every person was at risk of being found and afflicted. The truth is that the lack of sunlight made them depressed and the combination of rotten mutton, or dried and preserved meat usually mixed with berries, pushed the people who lived much of the year in darkness, over the edge. Anyone who has lived through a severe winter or two can tell stories of the depression, loneliness, and despair that can cover you if you do not take care in putting yourself out in the sun, taking herbal supplements, such as St. John's Wart and sour cherry juice, and focusing on distractions from the depression. It was growing up in the Northwest near the Seattle area that taught me about the importance of sunlight. Year after year, a sadness and slowing would come. At first, it was a gentle hibernation and creative stage, an acceptance of the rain and cool after the hot summer months. An excitement about the holidays prevails and then a dip so low it reflects the sugar high I had from Thanksgiving to Christmas. A pattern was born. By February of every year the depression and introversion was enough to drive anyone mad and then ahhhhh! SPRING!

Light therapy is very helpful in the production of serotonin or the chemical that promotes the healthy transfer of an electrical charge or pulse through the neurotransmitters, which control the healthy function of the body. The Sun provides humans and all living organisms with the right amount of UV light for their systems to create the vitamin D to support healthy function. The Sun is our natural battery charger and this is why over- exposure can zap you out or cause an irregular mutation and movement within the cells that can cause skin cancer. Our nervous system is the battery and the sun is the energy that keeps the neurotransmitters firing in rhythm. If this rhythm is disturbed the whole system is disturbed, resulting in an indefinite imbalance usually beginning in an already compromised area in the endocrine system that eventually affects the immune system.

The order in which light absorption affects the body as a system is as follows, the sequence is optic nerve (the receiver)—hypothalamus (the SCN, rhythm keeper and processor)—nervous system (the conductor)—endocrine system (the producer)—immune system (an effected system) and so forth. Light is one of the main components that keep the oscillating rhythm of our bodies in motion. Without the Sun's light in particular, everything of the Earth would lose the electrical charge controlling it's individual biorhythms and within days the entire clock/magnetism of the Earth would be affected.

The positive influence that light has on every living organism is a magnetic charge and the creation of vitamin D within the system once it has been touched by the sunlight. All it takes to activate the molecules of any kind of matter is the correct frequency of light. Sunlight is a necessary staple for cells of any kind to continue in homeostasis. Without it, all life would eventually disappear from our planet.

Five

Color

"Sound, light, vibration, and the form blend and merge, and thus the work is one.

It preceedeth under the law and naught can hinder now the work from going foreword.

The man breathes deeply. He concentrates his forces, and drives the thought from him."

THE CREATIVE WORK OF SOUND. THE SCIENCE OF BREATH. BY: ALICE E.

BAILY.

Color is the visible part of light gauged on the spectrum of electro-magnetic radiation. Most light is seen as white light and does not appear colored until it is split into the seven colors that make up the rainbow spectrum. Color travels in waves just like white light and is sensed by our eyes when those wavelengths hit our retina. Using color for healing purposes goes back in history a long way, Many books reference the famed "color halls" of ancient China, Egypt and India. After creating the color wheel, Sir Isaac Newton matched music notes to the different colors of the color spectrum finding similarities in their vibrations and became one of the most ingenuitive manipulators of color. Niels Finson made landmark discoveries concerning the anti-bacterial properties of ultra-violet light and found that he could reduce scarring of the skin with the healing properties of infrared. Johann Goethe was fascinated with the psychological affects of color on his clients. All of these men are fathers of color therapies in modern times.

It is simple to use color for healing. Students of color therapy are amazed when they begin to use color topically, finding that amazing results accompany their experiments. Every time I used the blue, clear, and violet light at the brow line or the location of the SCN, the main circadian rhythm center in the body, my clients would tell me that they felt tingling, warmth, and other pleasant feelings associated with the light. Chinese doctors believe that each part of the body needs to keep a certain temperature or vibration. The Chakras hold the vibration and color that affect and echo the energy levels of our organs and all the systems of the body. Therefore, we will focus on affecting the body as a whole through the chakras. We will focus on providing our bodies with the energy it needs to stay within the cycle of health. We can use the skin/integumentary system, optic nerves, and the entirety of the nervous system to affect our physical health. This only takes finding a safe color supply to use. The most effective way is to use daylight and color shields. Color shields should be created as transparent as possible using clear plastic. For example, find a room in your house where sunlight spills through the window. You can purchase a variety of saran wraps at any grocery store, green, yellow, purple, blue, pink, orange, etc. Try to fashion this wrap directly onto your window one color at a time. Stretch out in front of it and see how it makes you feel. Try cutting circles of color to fashion on your window and match them up with your chakras. Add aromas and music and now you have a healing sanctuary.

I like the idea of using natural means of light as you are healing within an area that is not being affected by a circuit of electricity. Many people like different colored light bulbs, try them, and see what you think. I personally have become fond of a tool created by the Colour Energy Corporation called *The Chromalive Light Pen.* It comes with seven removable, colored, crystal disc lenses. I use this in conjunction with crystal healing and in particular with the diamonds, which I will talk more about throughout the book. I have had an amazing response from people, usually a notable vibration accompanied by a sense of well being or release. The change in energy is near immediate. This pen uses a battery, which makes it nice for travel, but ranges in price of $500-800. Less expensive techniques should be used until you are comfortable and decide you like to use light as a means for healing.

Barbara Brennan, a well-known healer and atmospheric physicist, believes that both therapist and client must learn to feel what it is like to be in all of the colors, not just visualize them. It has been said by many that **energy follows thought**, and as we visualize all things, including color, the energy that radiates from within us and surrounds us without begins to change frequencies as they resonate within a particular color.

This is like blending colors within the color wheel, searching for the right resonance to be found within the color that flows with the rest of the picture. We learn to tune our color and help others to tune theirs. This means lying in a room full of one color will help you to learn what it means to be *in* a certain color and in this way, you can help to hold this feeling and transfer it to your clients. "I have found that color in the aura is directly related to sound. Sounding specific pitches into the field not only produces specific colors in the field, but is also a powerful agent for healing," Brennan states in her renowned book, *Hands of Light*. This is another example of how healers are matching sound to color and healing.

Six

The use of sound and vibrational healing

Musical instruments and the voice act as vibrational tools that can have an array of effects on the body. Musical orchestrations of all types have been tested for years. Most people have heard that people study better while listening to classical music, sleep better while listening to single instruments like the piano, flute, or harp, and get "amped" up while listening to upbeat music like rock or metal.

Music ignites visions, emotion, and passion within the listener and seems to make an impression on the mood. I do not believe that anyone needs a scientific explanation for this. In the case of healing with sound, each chakra/circadian rhythm center gives off a vibration that is affected by concentrated tone. One can help tune the chakra/SCN by singing or playing an instrument near the energy center. This is much like a music instructor clapping his hands or tapping his foot to help keep a student in rhythm. If the healing practitioner can apply heat, light, a gem, tuning forks, or direct manipulation in the form of massage/acupuncture to the area it will activate or polarize the molecules in ways that prepare the body for healing. Throughout the book, you may notice that I group words like energy center, oscillator, circadian, and SCN together, this is because I believe that these terms represent one system working in synchronicity. In the case of the human body, I believe that the chakras are visual representations of the oscillation or rhythm present in the site of a minor circadian or the bio-rhythmic keeper, the SCN (supra-chiasmatic nuclei).

Music helps to bring harmony among the energy of a chakra by helping to create order among disturbed or blocked energy waves, life force, or *Ch'i* in the body. "All geographic places have their own **notes**, arising from their unique interplay of countless harmonic associations between rocks, trees, mountains, lakes, streams, valleys, and waterfalls. In some places, the amplitude of this note seems higher. When someone feels pulled to a certain place by a higher force, they are getting a message of their need to be activated in a certain way. If they can surrender to their intuition they are renewed, perhaps transformed (J.A. Swan, *Sacred Places*)".

The Law of Octaves teaches students of healing how to manage the physical vibrations that exist around us and harness them in the appropriate way to encourage healing. Like color and light, each tone holds a definite number of vibrations per second, which we have identified as the hertz vibration. If one sings or plays a note and they rise up one octave the vibration doubles. Each scale represents an octave. Musician and spiritual teacher Kay Gardner writes, "When moving from audible sound waves to the visible light waves that produce the color spectrum, we must jump forty octaves." Light and color are not audible, so most of us do not make the connection between light and sound. It is a progression and there is a connection. The colors that correspond to the musical notes are not definite, because there are innumerable shades and hues available. But we know the basics and the basics are very useful when conducting a color and light therapy treatment. (Please see Ch. 9 on Chakras)

Music helps to fill a space, to balance/or imbalance a vibration. While working with my teacher, Sisiwin Lummi medicine man, Beaver Chief, I learned that vibration had always been used to create wellness where there had once been imbalances. He called the bell the new medicine and the drum the old medicine. When I would come to him with an ailment or a concern, he would use the vibration of his drum and voice to do the healing work. Beaver Chief would also place large crystals right on the body in an area that was out of balance and drum and sing only inches from the area. This was an amazing vibration to experience. He explained this by saying, "the drumming is the heartbeat of the Earth and aids me in connecting with the spirit world". He was physically removing blockages from my body and tuning the subtle forces that move within me with the power of strong vibration. I always experienced immediate results.

One experience in particular is always at the front of my mind when giving an example. Before I knew that I was experiencing a hormone imbalance due to poly-cystic-ovarian syndrome, I would sometimes go for up to four months without having a monthly cycle. I was 19 and worried that something was wrong. So, I went to Beaver Chief and told him my concerns and he told me that this was indeed an easy fix. He put me on a table face up, placed a fist-sized amethyst on my belly, and began to drum and sing directly at the crystal with his drum almost touching me. He did this for about 5 minutes. Within fifteen minutes, I had to use the rest room and to my delight and for a lack of better words, the blockage moved and I was indeed in flow. If a girl's monthly cycle could be that off and be regulated through rhythm and song so quickly, I definitely believe that the cancer patients he helped to recover over months of treatments were genuine healings. I met some of these people who were living radiant and healthy lives and are a true testimony to the benefits of alternative and faith healers.

Crystal bowls or singing bowls have a firm place in healing. Their size, width, and substance depict their sound. If you have ever been in a room with these bowls, you know they can change your mood quite quickly. I have gone from being alert and energetic, to wanting to take a nap. I have been in a punchy kind of a mood and after spinning a bowl left the area feeling calm and happy. This again, is very individual and the affects that these bowls and their powerful notes have are different from person to person. Some may feel a calming; others may get sick depending on what their body needs. A nauseating feeling often means that the vibration is more than what is needed, at the time.

A didgeridoo is a long hollow tube that usually becomes gradually wider at the bottom. This is a wind instrument that creates an incredible musical atmosphere and many people have told me stories of increased well being after having the didgeridoo blown around them in an intentional way. I would explain it by saying it creates an unreal feeling of being surrounded by sound and its varying vibrations.

Once again, sound is affecting the movement of every cell in your body. Certain regulating sounds, like that of a singing bowl, or a steady note on a flute, can help to set your energy in alignment. This means the cells move in a more orderly fashion, getting to their destinations more effectively. Sound vibration provides a kind of trail map for our cells. Our cells always get where they should go eventually because of the constant pumping of the heart. They just bump around a little bit more. A visual example of this would be a trickling stream where the water meanders gently stopping to swirl and caress the rocks in a mild fashion. If the floodgates open, there is more energy and momentum moving the water forward above the rocks and swirls within the current, making it easier for the water to meet its destination. Sound vibration can be an amazing tool for healing, indeed.

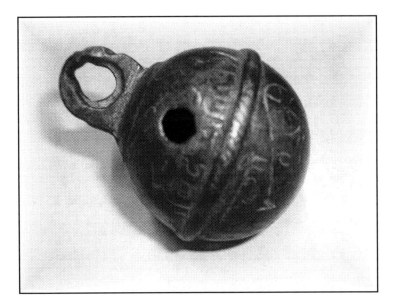

Brass Bell

What happens if I am musically disabled?

"We human beings don't just enjoy music, all our physiology, its rhythms and interactions, follow the laws of music."

Mary Theines-Schunemann, composer and music educator

In truth, not all people are born with the genes of Mozart running through their veins. I have tried many times to play all kinds of musical instruments and over many years I have found that in order to play really well I would need to seek out lessons. The good news is you do not have to play really well, to create the vibration needed for healing. Singing bowls are an easy tool to use if one can hold their hand steady and keep a hold on the wrapped handle. Bongo drumming can be extremely rhythmic and healing and you don't have to be able to hold a super creative beat to use the drum. It is only necessary to keep the *wom wom wom wom* beat to create a field of vibration suitable for healing. I cannot explain the ways the vibration of a simple note creates an opening or a kind of allowance for healing to happen in a sacred space. Again, this is individual; some people need certain notes for tuning their bodies and don't need others. Nausea, headache, vertigo, and anxiety are all signs of an over-reaction within the individual. Peace, relaxation, and general wellbeing are obvious signs that the right notes and tunes are being performed. I suggest choosing a simple pipe flute, a nice flat drum with a wrapped handle, a rattle or singing bowls. These are effective and strong instruments and perfect for the musical novice.

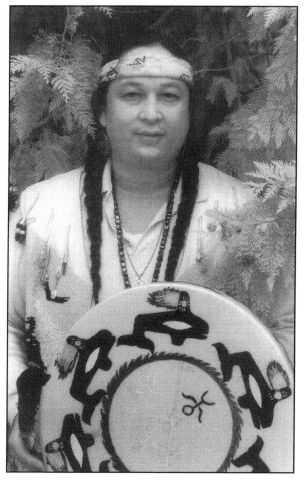

Beaver Chief with drum   January 15, 1955-June 8, 2001

Seven

Aromatherapy

The benefits found by those who use aroma as therapy should be considered proof that nature provides all of the answers. Aroma is a link to memory and memory creates patterns. As a whole, the cultures of the world have done a good job of discovering some of the mysteries of our Earth as well as our universe. Nutrients provided to us in nature are the keys to health. Balance within our diets may not be able to bring us out of disease all on its own, but a combination of supplements, tonics, teas, aromas, body cleansing, and diet can make a life changing impression on those who are serious about their health. Much of this comes from their intention to be healthy, this means to be as clean as possible mentally and physically. David Crow is a celebrated aroma therapist and licensed acupuncturist. He has traveled the world to help create sustainable healthcare and economies, as well as ecological restoration and preservation through the utilization and education of medicinal plants.

"Essential oils have a direct and profound effect on the deepest levels of the body and psyche. Because their primary route of absorption is inhalation, they have a strong and immediate influence on the mucous membranes of the respiratory system. Passing through the capillary beds of the sinuses and activating the olfactory nerves, the fragrances of the oils enter the brain, producing systemic effects on the neurological, immunological, and hormonal functions. Essential oils powerfully enhance positive mental and emotional states, and build resistance to pathogens," says David Crow.

Separating the physical substance of any kind of flora creates aromas. Just like all organisms, plants are a product of their environment. That is why we live at such an opportune time to be healthy. We can experiment with different plants, vitamins, and mineral supplements found all over the world. Aroma and essential oils are processed with greater ease by the body than a pharmaceutical drug. A drug enters the body through the blood stream, affecting every organ directly. Once processed by the body, it can take weeks to process a drug out. This creates a reaction of health or disharmony depending upon the individual. The body reacts to aroma in a subtle way. Do you sneeze or do you feel immediately drawn in by a deep breath as you experience one of these gentle elements of nature? Your subtle reactions lets you know if you need them or not. Does the smell put you off or give you a headache? On the other hand, does this smell remind you of something positive, comforting, familiar, and relaxing?

Why does the public reduce themselves into ignorance by passively using pharmaceuticals? If something gives you diarrhea, headache, nervousness, sleeplessness, or loss of interest in the world around you, ask yourself, do you trust this drug to heal you, to mend you, to bring balance into your already disrupted system we call our body? I hope not. I am not suggesting that aromas and other supplements should be used to fight all ailments; I am suggesting that the public has a wealth of supplements that grow in the natural environment and when consumed in the right way, in the right amount, and for the right reasons, can be used as a tool for healing.

People who are experts on the intake of aroma are called aroma-therapists. These people are very helpful to those who have very little experience with aroma and other essences. One must always be conscious of toxicity, balance, and health. This is an individual matter and has a lot to do with a person's biological make-up and personal history.

While performing any kind of bodywork, I have found it incredibly beneficial to use aromas to encourage positive visualizations and to induce comfort. Scent has a strong affect on the memory and most people have vivid visualizations or other sensations that correspond with the smell. It is very important to create an environment for yourself and your clients that will feel healing and nurturing. Aromatherapy provides the body with the information it needs to relax just by offering a pleasant smell, and helps the client trust and open for the sake of healing. The respiratory system controls the amount of oxygen we let into our blood streams. If we inhale mustard gas, our respiratory system reacts as if it is under attack. Mucus spills from every orifice and all of the blood rushes to the inflicted organs, which help us to expel this poison from our systems. Yet, if one already has a bronchial infection and cannot sleep, eat, or breathe comfortably, a mustard seed oil or ground mustard seed compress can be applied to the chest with the olfactory drawing the aroma into the body and aiding the respiratory system in its natural process of achieving balance. A controlled amount of a known noxious substance is not only harmless in this case, but a helpful remedy. This can be the means to recovery.

Our stomachs and intestines are meant for processing bulk amounts of nutrients like meats, veggies, nuts, seeds, herbs, and berries. It can only process what you consume and if you consume too much your body will drive out the toxic levels quickly, sometimes making one expel it violently. An over consumption of processed and additive rich foods can also be very difficult and disruptive during digestion. An additive is something added to a food, which is not normally present in its natural form. A general rule can be followed here, the more additives one consumes, the more you have added to your body's difficult toxin eliminating process. Additives are not supposed to be there. In small amounts the body can deal with them, in large amounts, the body begins to over-work and eventually will fall into dysfunction. In the same way that we choose foods that are fresh, nourishing, and organic if possible, I encourage you to use the purest of aroma and essential oils for the purpose of healing yourself and others.

Aromatherapy is an important tool. It helps to bring a subtle balance to the body, much like music and color. Aromas like any medicinal should be used with care. The following aroma oils are essential buys when building a starter aromatherapy kit.

Cedarwood: It is a powerful antiseptic and can be used to draw out toxins from the skin and helps to break down mucus. It is deep, earthy and rich. Warms the home and mood while bringing the essence of the outdoors, inside.

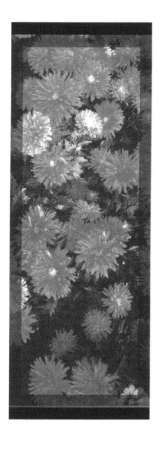

Orange: Is a stimulant to the lymph and digestive systems. Can also be used as a sedative for anxiety, sleeplessness and can calm heart palpitations. Oranges have a positive and lightening effect on the mood.

Clove: Can have a numbing effect like an analgesic if used in small amounts on the gums during a toothache or teething. Works as an aphrodisiac. Can be used as a stimulant and an antiseptic.

Rose: A powerful anti-depressant. Helps treat disorders of the female reproductive system. Calms the mind.

Eucalyptus: Is best known for it's anti-viral and anti-septic. Opens and clears the sinuses and the lungs. Can be used as a compress on bug bites or scratches.

Lavender: Has been used to stimulate paralyzed limbs. It heals burns, helps bruising and stretch marks. It is a good decongestant and helps people to sleep peacefully. Place at the temples during migraines/headaches.

Ylang-ylang: Has a regulating affect on the nervous system and encourages hair growth. An exotic euphoric scent.

Sage: Considered a sacred plant, the oil can be mixed with water to clear the whole Aura. Used in poultices & gargles.

Rosemary: Also a sacred plant, helps to cure nervous disorders, hair loss, circulation, helps digestion, over-exertion, and pain

Eight

The Control Cycle

Ki is the word that represents both breath and the vital life force in both the Japanese and Chinese cultures. Ki/Ch'i/Qi are all words that explain the universal force that drives life through our bodies. It is the physical conduction of the pulse. It is this Ki that keeps the cycles of control and generation in motion.

The real ideal is that each system and organ of the body relies on the health in balance of all of the systems. When you study the control cycle and the natural direction of the five points of the star, it is easy to relate the organs to one another. Disease and malfunction are the result of an organ or a system having an imbalance. If there is an imbalance in one system, it will show up in another system. Maybe the circulatory system needs more oxygen, perhaps the liver needs more water, and the muscles may need more potassium. Whatever the need, the eventual depletion of Ch'i or life force causes malfunction to be visible in the body. If circulation is low because of dehydration, it is only a matter of time before a real imbalance is recognized. If the body is low on anti-oxidants, the body will present minor problems that add up over time and will call for balance to be regained in all of the systems of the body. Massage and acupuncture help to bring circulation into areas of the body that have become oxygen or Chi deficient. These methods of healing awaken the body and prepare the cells to absorb nutrients again. Eastern practitioners talk about energy blocks and the meridians. A perfect example of "toxins" being stored, built up, or "blocked" within the body is found in the case of gout. Gout is the result of our blood stream not cleaning itself properly and moment by moment, the toxins are deposited in areas of low circulation within the body like the extremities. In theory, it would seem appropriate to have an enema, drink some sour cherry juice along with a detoxifying tea for a day or two, and then have a massage or an acupuncture session that focuses on circulating the blood, relieving the damaged tissue. It is common knowledge that just drinking water can help to flush the body on its own. What systems have been affected? The lungs need more oxygen rich breath, the heart needs more clean oxygenated blood, the liver needs more space to work the toxins out into the kidneys that have to be clean enough to filter correctly to the bladder. Eventually, all of this will affect the nervous system, which is usually where people begin to identify pain with imbalance. Because Eastern medicine works to treat the whole body, rather than a symptom or a localized area, work needs to be done on some level with integration and focus on all of the parts creating the whole. Modalities of Western thought tend to look at the curative process in a linear way, going from A to B to C. Eastern modalities have a circulatory approach regarding the body as a whole mechanism that must be treated as a completely rounded system, not in pieces. Though infinitely varied, everything in the universe is connected. Therefore, to regain health out of disease one must work on the diet, their outside and internal environments, and the health of the mental, physical, and spiritual aspects in a way that makes one more whole.

This is a brief description of the control cycle that will help every practitioner of the healing arts on their theory and order of treatment. I suggest reading *Fusion of the Five Elements 1,* by Mantak Chia and *The Book of Shiatsu*, by Paul Lundberg. Lundberg has a great way of simplifying information and Mantak Chia has an amazing theory for an advancing student.

Nine

The Chakras

The first mention of a Chakra was found in the written text of the Vedas. The Vedas (2,000-600 BC) are the oldest written tradition in India. The word Chakra means "wheel" and is a metaphor for the sun. The Yoga Upanishads (600 AD) tell of the chakras being centers of psychic consciousness. In 200 BC, the Yoga Sutra of Patanjali talks of the dualities of the physical, spiritual, and natural world. In 1919, a man by the name of Arthur Avalon translated the texts Sat-Cakra-Nirupana, Padaka-Pancaka, and Gorakshashatakam. His book is called *The Serpent Power* and includes meditations, explanations, and descriptions of the chakras.

Almost all of the spiritual practices that claim to help people physically acknowledge one of the following: spirit/spirits, energy, chakras, and auras. It is simple to accept these ideas when we understand how the spirit energy is produced and how we are directly affected by it.

I am including many references in this book to aid the reader in sourcing valuable references that give all kinds of historical and differentiating viewpoints.

The most common definition for a chakra goes something like this: A chakra is one of seven main energy centers in the body. A chakra emits energy that is read vibrationally by its color and sometimes tone. Each of the seven chakras directly relates to an area of the body marked by a clump of nerve related tissue, organs, glands, hormones, and or an emotion. These chakras can help a healing practitioner work through many disorders with a client. Professionals in the field of energy work use the color of the chakra as a guide to understanding an imbalance in the body. Many see the chakras as moving, spinning, or fanning places of energy. This makes sense, because our cells move naturally in a circling motion and as energy follows the same pattern, our chakras move in the way of the circle. If one observes a faint coloration or no color in the area of one of the chakras, this is a sign that there is dysfunction in the way of blocked or low energy in the correlating areas of the body. A difference in temperature in the air around the client or even on the surface of the skin can also give indications of excessive or low energy within the client's physical and/or spiritual body. When working with the chakras, each one has a different way of showing imbalance. The person doing the energy work can usually pick up on visual, emotional, physical and sometimes olfactory and audio based information that is being held in the body.

There are many different modalities of healing which depend on the information collected so far about how the chakras work. Most people recognize fields like Reiki, healing touch, yoga, shiatsu, and acupuncture. A new field of bio-energy workers are being born with the rise in demand for options within the healing arts. I am recognizing a need to clarify a place where the words begin to blur for some and for those who are interested in receiving or practicing a healing art.

I find that knowing the qualities of the chakras help to define their purpose and their meaning within the field of healing and learning to heal ourselves.

1ˢᵗ chakra
Root chakra
Red
Musical note: C
Vibrates @261.1 cycles/second
Will to live, grounding, physical vitality
Adrenal glands, metabolism, sexual vitality, bony structure of the spine

3ʳᵈ chakra
Solar Plexus
Yellow
Musical note: E
Vibrates @329.1 cycles per/sec
Receives healing energy for meditation and sends out energy for manifestation
Pancreas, liver, gall bladder, nervous system

5ᵗʰ chakra
Throat Chakra
Blue
Musical note: G
Vibrates @392 cycles per/sec
Communication, sound, expression on all levels
Thyroid, lungs, voice box, throat

2ⁿᵈ chakra
Sacral chakra
Orange
Musical note: D
Vibrates @292.1 cycles/sec
Creativity, courage, self-esteem, emotions
Gonads/Ovaries, reproductive and digestive systems

4ᵗʰ chakra
Heart Chakra
Pink/Green
Musical note: F
Vibrates @349.2 cycles per/sec
Center of compassion, love, and group consciousness
Thymus, Heart, blood, circulatory system

6ᵗʰ chakra
Third eye chakra
Indigo/violet
Musical note: A
440 cycles per/sec
Psychic guidance, intuition, magnetic energy,
light energy, the unknown
Pituitary gland, hypothalamus, sensory organs, nervous system

7ᵗʰ chakra
Crown
White/golden
Musical note: B
493 cycles per/sec
Purity, connects to god-energy, divine consciousness, enlightenment, dynamic thought
Pineal gland, divine energy

Barbara Brennan is a scientist and a healer. In her book, *Hands of Light*, she gives a wonderful breakdown of the ways a practitioner of the healing arts perceives information that is being held within the chakras. I have used this insight as an effective guide for my own path and involvement within the healing arts.

Brennan reminds bodyworkers to be very aware, allowing your clients body to send all of the subtle information it can to be felt out by our receivers, the chakras. Brennan suggests that our chakras each have a different kind of sensory information that can be detected through each individual chakra.

The first chakra detects movement, balance, and kinesthetics. This chakra allows you to feel sympathetic pains and illness. Such as neck pain that has no apparent root in yourself, but seems to be a replication of the woman's whiplash injury that you worked on in the morning. As bodyworkers, we wash our hands and energetically clear ourselves automatically after each client. We do this not only for the sake of germs, but also because we must make an energetic break between our clients and ourselves. It can be interesting at first to experience residual feelings or images left behind by our clients, but after some time this will impact our own physiological and spiritual selves, mostly in undesirable ways. Water is an element that is naturally clearing and renewing physically and spiritually.

The second chakra provides emotional information connected to health and injury. Physically we relate this in the form of clenching fists, unhealthy holding patterns from pain and anxiety, or the spiritual and mental cutting off of an injured area. All of these physical symptoms are ourselves holding emotional reactions. We know that muscle tissue holds memory. We must not only be aware of this, but prepared to work with this if the situation arises. It can be rewarding to work with a client who has gone through cancer, has been battered, or is working through depression. One can feel an unraveling when a connection is made and when one feels safe enough to let go of their pain, anger, or sadness associated with a physical or mental and always emotional issue. I have been known to cry a lot during or after a session, feel downtrodden, confused, or anxious. All of this because I connected deeply to the emotion within them, I guided them through an unraveling and did not disconnect myself properly and fully from them when the session was over. We learn to do this out of necessity and over time.

The solar plexus provides the gut feelings that come on sometimes very strongly and sometimes very vaguely. These are the feelings that make one take the back roads home, avoiding an accident, or urges one to say something nice to someone who just found out about the death of a loved one. If one communicates with or observes the spirit world, this is the chakra that alerts one of the kind of presence that is there.

The fourth chakra provides the receiver with feelings of love and compassion. This chakra is the most easily activated in the healer and student of healing, as well as the most easily knocked out of balance. This chakra gives more that any other; it influences our actions, thoughts, and guides our hearts to do what work is truly needed to begin the process of balance in others and ourselves. Have you ever listened to a song that reaches right into your soul and plucks the strings of emotion that cause images to spin in your head, tears to flow from your eyes, and leaves you with a feeling like you've awaken from a dream of deep love and knowing? This is the heart chakra reacting.

The fifth chakra receives information in clear verbal messages. This chakra communicates messages in the ways of sound, smell, and taste. Some people see full visual information, much like the work of Edgar Cayce. Edgar Cayce, in my opinion, is one of the most important people to study to learn about hypnosis bringing information through for the practitioner and the client to work with. I do not receive very much in full sentences; I receive words, which is usually enough. On the dark slate of my mind, I will see the word *tennis*, and at that moment, my hands are spreading a tough bicep muscle. I can then see the person taking a swing at a ball, and very quickly my mind zooms into the shoulder and I am able to see the cause and remedy of a particular structural imbalance. This is actually the fifth and sixth chakras working together to provide a clear glimpse into injury and solution.

The sixth chakra is the chakra of hunches and psychic thought, so this is a visual chakra through which we can receive information. One may see the situation that caused an injury, or the exact place that needs the pressure or circulation to cause an initial opening for the relief of pain or suffering. This chakra fills the screen in your mind. This chakra requires a person to be very open allowing for unopinionated images to form.

The seventh chakra will reveal a glimpse into the life path of the person. These are the lessons or changes that the injury caused that were necessary for the person in this life. Some call this karma. These are the injuries and illnesses that are only remedied when the client is ready to fix them. We are never in control of the path of another person and it is important to accept these limitations. If we confront them and try to make changes that are not ours to make at the time, we will find ourselves drained and eventually ill. In the same way, we can be guides for our clients, offering them information that will lead them forward on their path towards healing. Pay attention.

Ten

Circadian Rhythms and the SCN

Most people relate chakras with the aura. The two indeed do work together directly. It has been documented that genuine energy workers and intuitive healers are somehow able to focus on areas of their patient's bodies that scientifically prove dysfunction. This is the place where science and spirit meet. It is a great time we live in and the information that I am sharing is relative as well as useful for the people who are stepping into the field of healing. Most people do not know that all of the systems in our bodies are controlled by a mechanism located in the hypothalamus just above the optic chiasm called the SCN or the suprachiasmatic nuclei. Most people are more familiar with the term biorhythm or an intrinsically patterned cyclical and biological function inherent to all life. Just like a car needs a timing belt so everything happens rhythmically when it should, your body needs something that keeps it running smoothly as well. The SCN works with the hypothalamus and the optic nerve to create an environment within the body that is conducive to life. This is done by taking in sunlight and using it as energy and information for the body. At the same time, the pineal gland is located in the hypothalamus above the third ventricle and is affected in every way by the intake of sunlight. This is the part of the brain where sunlight is processed and used to regulate cycles in the body, such as melatonin for sleep. The SCN is a natural pacemaker for the body, because it keeps its own beat or rhythm. This beat is different from the most well known biorhythm, the heartbeat. It holds more of a pulsating rhythm caused by the very movement of the body's cells. The hypothalamus relates to the SCN in the way that both seem to have a controlling influence over the functioning of hormones, body temperature, water balance, sleep cycles, control of appetite, and any emotion involved in causing pleasure, fear, anger, sexual arousal, and pain.

"The SCN are able to generate rhythms on their own without any light cues. Under normal operations however, the SCN are synchronized with the day-night cycle of their surroundings, the entrainment paths being visual projections directly from the retina. In fact, it has very recently been discovered that the eye contains special photo-sensors, not used for vision, connected directly to the SCN, enabling people who are blind to entrain their circadian rhythms."

People are taking in sunlight to nourish and tune the systems of the body, even though they cannot see it. We do not need sight to feel the Sun charging our bodies and filling them with the energy needed to keep our bodies healthy. Just go take a little nap out in the sunshine and see how you feel!

"Many separate circadian oscillators have now been found scattered through out the body, to regulate local rhythms in behavior and physiological functioning. These timers can maintain their rhythms by themselves for only a few days and are constantly entrained by signals from the master clock, the SCN".(Roger Newton, *Galileo's Pendulum*)

The SCN keeps something called a circadian rhythm, which means it moves in a spiraling like movement that is created by the natural oscillation, movement or rhythm of every cell within its designated clump of nervous tissue. If you could imagine a single cell in a pitre dish that you could track over a 24-hour time period, you would find that the cell would have strategically drawn a spiraling shape through its naturally rhythmic movement. This spiral is the framework of our energetic body. The rhythm is caused by the cells natural movement through the body and their atomic interaction with all of the other cells in the body through their inherent electrical nature. The SCN at the hypothalamus is the regulating center of rhythm by which the other minor SCN or circadians set their beats to and machine and man read their circulating energy in varying color or hertz vibrations. Each color carries a varying amount of hertz energy.

What does this mean? It is my belief that the SCN, which depends upon our optic nerve's ability to receive light and communicates the data to the hypothalamus for use by the nervous system and endocrine systems for cyclical regulation corresponds directly to the system of chakras that was introduced to the world thousands of years ago in the Eastern civilizations, specifically in India. It means that we have something concrete to base our ideas on when we are conducting healing for our clients. Our chakras can act like a built in energy gauge for our bodies if we learn to use tools like the pendulum to read their rhythms and frequencies. Holding color for a client and working to improve their energetic life force becomes more than a simple visualization practice; it is much more like tuning a fine instrument. The Colour Energy Co. reminds me that the German physicist Dr. Fritz-Albert Popp proved that the cells of all living beings emit "biophotons" (light quanta). This radiation represents a regulating energy field, which influences the total biochemical processes inside of us. All forces are explained in quanta, except for gravity, presenting a manifestation of fields of energy. All quanta are represented by the same mathematic mechanism, based on their oscillation or ability to hold vibration through controlled movement. The idea I would like to present is that we can tune our circadians using light, amplify the light using diamonds, and enhance the whole process by providing specific colors that our bodies need and use to stay within health. Our health and imbalances are mirrored in our biofield, making the work we do on the physical body through various forms of bodywork and the work we do on the internal body through diet, exercise activities, and supplements, just as important as energy work and diagnosis using tuning and healing tools. Integration of all these facets of health is making an approach to wholeness. The chakras, hormonal glands, nerves and the suprachiasmatic nuclei (SCN) represent every system in the body. The SCN gives a facilitator of healing the ability to perceive the varied energies and energy centers of the body. Visually, we are able to perceive the varying light waves and vibrations through differentiating color. The SCN and the chakras work as one in the same way the bio-field and the oscillatory vibration creating any field of color is one. What creates the energy and color held in each chakra are the varying vibrational energies caused by the oscillating movement of the cells that exist in the clumps of nervous tissue scattered through out the body regulating function in all that one can imagine possible. For example, the reason the root chakra is red is because it is a colorful manifestation of the rhythmic pulse being exuded from the electrical quality of the nerve plexus closest to it.

One must realize that we are working with the energy that resides within the organ or system of the body that we want to affect. Through all of the explanations I have given, what I hope to provide is knowledge about how to make this energy tangible to the practitioners, so that they can incorporate it into their practice. We can create health in a client by helping the body to create a healing environment for it to regulate its own systems. We do this by helping the nervous system to release from any impingements or blockages, through hot and cold therapies, full body integration therapies such as massage or yoga. These techniques aid, balance, and calm the muscular systems. We prepare the circulatory system along with all other systems in the same way, with breathing, holistic therapies, and physical exercise. The whole body brought into wholeness. However, if one does not truly understand what they are working with, how can true balance be accomplished? Aroma, music, natural light, and an atmosphere of serenity are key in creating a safe environment that promotes emotional balance and support for the client. Acupuncture, massage, diet, and herb consultation all help to bring the physical into balance during a therapy session. Education and understanding of the physiological and energetic aspects of the body are essential to providing aid to a person who is dealing with imbalances and illness.

The SCN and Chakra system are the key locations that regulate the physical and spiritual energy of our bodies. I believe that a holistic approach that integrates both science and the art of healing is the preferred direction for healthcare in our future. The SCN in particular helps us to make a tangible connection between both areas of study.

Eleven

Auras

The aura is a recognized field of energy that exists around any living organism. The depth of an organism's aura depends on the vibration of its elemental molecular structure. When a cell vibrates, it produces thermal energy. People who study the science of cellular biology understand that when a cell of any kind dies it leaves behind a byproduct of some sort. Many people believe that energy never dies; it only changes its form. Anthropologists use this same process to determine how long ago a wooden tool fell to the ground or how many generations of people lived in the same area by testing materials found in archaeological sites, like fire pits, for example.

The most common form of evaluation is called carbon 14 dating. As a material decays and becomes a part of the earth again, its cellular structure changes, emits radiation and the elements that used to hold the material or organism together transform into other elements naturally. It is the same way in the bodies of human beings. Each food we digest, each pharmaceutical drug we take, each skin care product we use all have a natural process of decay. Our bodies are decaying each day and the only thing that slows this decay is the way we choose to live our lives day by day. If we abuse our body by forcing it to process toxic elements and chemicals of any amount the cells, mechanisms, and eventually organs in our body will process the sludge more slowly and eventually have so little energy left to use that they will shut down. This is the basis of all life. Over thousands of years, any organism can evolve to tolerate different toxic or unlivable influences in order for the genus to survive. Breeds that are more tolerant will have a higher survival rate. Yet, if too much stress is put on any group or individual over time, no matter how tolerant, the organism will shut down, become diseased, and die.

How does this relate to the aura or the human biofield? We have already established that thermal energy is measured in color or hertz vibration. Every part of the body needs to keep a balance of energy in it that helps it to be advantageous in supporting its relating systems and for the continuation of healthy living. When a practitioner of the healing arts is reading your "aura," what they are doing is tapping into your true vibration. If you are sick, it will show in your biofield and the same if you are healthy. If you are nervous, angry, or confused your heart beat rises and energetically this can be seen as heat. If you are on anti-depressants, alcohol, or cocaine, generally this will slow down the natural processes of most of your body while demanding a larger amount of blood for use around the kidneys and liver to process these chemicals. People who are diagnosing the aura in order to help an individual bring balance to the body are recognizing these patterns and helping people to focus on their bodies as a whole. The chakras define the bio-field by giving us a basic table of reference to what the normal levels of energy are in different areas and systems within the body.

Many people who have studied this field of alternative thought and medicine have found there to be between 7 to 9 different magnetic layers that make up the human aura or biofield. These layers also tend to have different colors attached to them. I like to reference William Wilks on this because I believe that he really has hit on something with his studies of magnetics during his years of retirement. During his study on the aura, he found that he could define each layer with a water-witching tool or an angle wire. He found that each layer of the aura had a sequential positive-negative-positive-negative charge and that the bio-field acts like a human atmosphere. Naturally, the aura repels what does not resonate with it and allows what has a neutral and/or positive reaction to give off no warning signal to the body. Each layer depends on the next for balance and support, so that if there is a disturbance in the third layer, the disturbance will be felt and will seek the means of balance from the surrounding layers.

Twelve

Earth Energy and the Biofield

Earth Energy is the same energy that people and animals feel when they visit an energy vortex or a place that is not favorable to the existence of life. I visited a vortex in Montana near Glacier Park with a good friend in 1999. We spent about an hour there. This striking experiment showed me just how our bodies give us telling signs on how we as individuals are reacting to the environment around us. We experimented with the valid presentation of backwards magnetics, various heightened gravity experiments, took lots of pictures that did not turn out at all and went on our way after I started experiencing dizziness and my stomach began to turn. This lasted for about an hour. My friend did not experience this at all, but was sympathetic to my sensitivity.

My body was sending me clear signals that whatever energy lived in the earth there was not healthy for me. This is all explainable. Native Americans have always considered these areas as cursed or sacred. No matter what the label, living organisms did not choose to make a home at these places on the earth. There were no Indian sacrifice ceremonies performed there that gave me a bad vibe, it was the magnetic ley lines, volcanic disturbances, and other unidentified mechanisms at work within our Earth that create such sites and humans have just recognized them.

I invite people to think about how they feel when they walk through a lava field or bathe in pure glacial water or in the ocean. How does it feel to sit outside during a lightning storm? You smell it and you feel it. I have watched the force of magnetics at work while hiking the "sliding sands" trail through Maui's volcanic Haleakala Crater. I sat down on a rock to take a rest and mindlessly began to stare at my footprints laid out before me. I noticed that the pebbles I had just walked on seemed to be sliding and moving naturally, yet noticeably filling the deepest area first and working its way until the footprint was an indistinct imprint. By the time I was done resting, the pebbles had all slid and moved erasing my footpath. Each pebble being made from the magma within the earth held a magnetic charge that moved until a polar balance among the particles was created.

When most people go for a day in the sun to a safe beach, they feel a general sense of well being. The sunlight encourages the production of serotonin helping all of the neuro-transmitters to fire in rhythm and the harmonizing ionic reaction that sea-water has on the make-up of our bodies is undeniably amazing and releasing. This is one of the reasons that one can find genuine sea salts in every spa and retail beauty store in America. Sea salts work to draw out toxins, create a neutralizing magnetic charge that helps to regulate all systems in the body, at the same time nourishing the skin. The positive result of eating Omega 3's, which are provided by all sea foods, have also directed our consciousness towards the creation of healthy stronger cell structures. I encourage everyone to consider blue-green algae, sea salts, and seafood if this resonates with them. All of the minerals and trace elements one needs to live a healthy life are found within the sea and the organisms that it supports.

We all know that we are drawn to different places to live and visit. We go to some places for pure pleasure, others to experience the pure mystery of the area. Sometimes we visit a place and just know something bad happened there. Overcome with anxiety or fear, we leave, not feeling safe. This reaction is due to our consciousness and our personal energy interacting with the energy held in the place. This is earth energy.

The make-up of our Earth and the unlimited amounts of healthy and unhealthy reactions that are created by elemental and chemical interactions directly affect every living organism. The Earth and its biofield influence us. At one time, the Earth had a natural way of influencing the very type of organism that could exist in a given place. Now, human beings being transient can alter this, sometimes successfully and many times unsuccessfully. Everything on the earth and within the Earth emits some amount of energy and collectively this creates the biofield of the Earth. This is a realm filled with electricity, magnetic forces, and light, among other types of energy, and it co-exists with the very air we breathe. This biofield holds the energy of everything that is and everything that was. It also holds the potential for everything that will ever be. This is why we experience the world of spirit. When the physical shell of our bodies no longer exists, the interactions and reactions that the life created can never be lost. Physical matter may decay, but it is used by another organism in some way and this is undeniable and unstoppable.

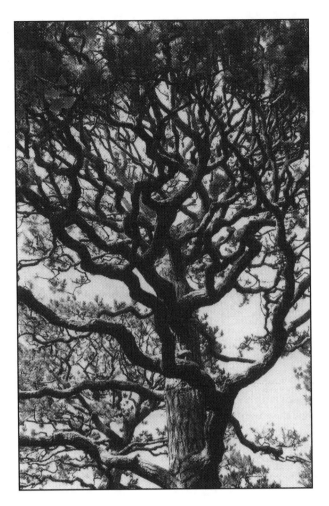

Tree of Life

Life becomes life becomes life. The physical is always recycled into all other matter on the planet and the essence is transferred through breakdown and decay. Because energy is the catalyst for life in matter, energy itself cannot die; it can change, but not die. Energy moves on with the recycling of physical matter.

Thirteen

The Pendulum

"…and yet it moves".

GALILEO

Galileo Galilei was just seventeen when he noticed the chandelier above him swaying ever so gently with the breeze. Timing the sway against the beat of his heart, he realized very quickly that there was no difference in the timing of its full swing from when it hardly swung at all, to when it swung in a slightly circular movement more widely. This type of rhythm keeping or oscillation was termed isochronism, having differentiating beats that keep the same timing. Pendulums are accepted as timekeepers mostly in clocks and in the new age world as divining devices. Through history, we have found that many of these rhythmic oscillations could manifest themselves in all kinds of natural phenomena. Today, the harmonic oscillator or Galileo's pendulum is much more than a timing device. Vibration moves us through life. "The phenomenon of natural oscillation has been found to be the basis of what we hear as sound, see as colors of light, and has helped us to understand the fabric of our universe through the quantum theory. Without oscillator's, there would be no particles, no air to breathe, and no solid matter to form the Earth" (Newton, Roger G., Galileo's Pendulum, 2004).

So far, science and the works of medicine have tangible, tested, and recorded bodies of evidence that one can depend upon and reference for answers. As for myself, a former student of the sciences, the healing arts has always been a form of science. This is why the pendulum is so interesting to me. I find that it is necessary to understand how things work if one wants to perform and participate in any field of interest. The field of healing just has more to it than many people had once assumed. In order to work on the body, a student is taught anatomy and physiology. This is a great start. Now, that each body part has an explanation, how do we as students, understand what controls the emotions, the spirit, or the quality of life of each individual who seem to have the same body parts? We must focus on what we all have in common, rather than concentrating on our varied spiritual beliefs that tend to tear us apart. The biggest thing that we have in common as humans is the energetic framework that we are made of and what everything is made of.

A traditional pendulum works by being an energetically sensitive device. The material it is made out of can be made from almost anything as long as the ratio of weight is distributed correctly. It is easy to create your own pendulum. Beading and jewelry making stores usually carry all of the supplies one needs. I prefer to use a semi-symmetrical natural crystal or gemstone that comes to a point at one end for a weight. The stone can be wrapped in any kind of metal wire and fastened to a chain or cord. A very lightweight chain or cord is preferable, because the weight should be heavier than the cord/chain. Find a small bead made of stone or metal material that you feel drawn to. This is the part of the pendulum that you will hold between you fingers. Cut a piece of wire from the same spool that you used to wrap the weight and push it through the beads hole. Use a pair of needle nose pliers to pinch off one end of the wire into a flattened head to hold the bead. Form the other end of the wire into a loop that you use to fasten to the cord or chain. Now, hold the bead between your thumb and pointer finger and feel the sway of the weight. Close your eyes and ask in your mind or out loud an obvious yes or no question like, "Is the Sun hot?" Watch the pendulum and be very still, notice the spin path that your weight begins to follow and know that this is the direction that your pendulum will move when it is responding to a question in which case the answer is, yes. This is your first pendulum.

The common belief is that each of us knows the answer to all of our quandaries within our own hearts and minds. The pendulum will pick up on the subtle electrical energy and vibrations we are sending out and that are being held within our personal biofield. Copper is a great conductor of this energy and I suggest using this metal to create your first pendulum.

In Native American Indian ideology, everything holds the energy of life. This includes the rocks, the water, the mountains, the animals, and everything that is apart of this earth. They call this energy mana or animism. Mana is the means by which they chose to describe the energy that moves the world around them. Christians call this the creative energy of God. The Chinese call it Ch'i, the Japanese call it Ki, Aborigine's from Australia call it djang, and the Hawaiian people see it as breath. America has a mixed culture that has allowed confusion, controversy, and sometimes acceptance in the case of spiritual matters and what drives the world around us. This sacred energy is the movement of life and the same energy that the pendulums recognize.

The big bang theory explains the combining and activation of molecules in our universe. Just as a crystal creates an electric current while under pressure, so it is the same with the massive rocks that float around in space that we call stars and planets. The possibilities for life are indeed endless. The colliding of mass on that scale is likened to an atomic blast, changing the energy that surrounds the collision indefinitely. As the waves of energy disperse from the pressure of the collision, the waves move through and have an effect on every molecule, changing them in one way or another. These are the same waves of energy that bring life to the molecules that move here on earth. Subtle changes occur in the molecules under the effect of the energy created by the collision. These subtle changes allow for new life forms to be created out of the residual debris and energy of such a collision. So, it seems that the mere pressure of two large inanimate rocks are able to create the energy that is needed to create the magnificence of life that has spawned on our planet. It is commonly known that pressure creates heat, sound, and a blast of light waves. I believe that this is the same energy that creates all life and all that is. Spirit is a combination of the three without a physical form that on the norm, we cannot see in our field of vision. It does not mean that it is not there or that it cannot exist, we just cannot touch it, because its form is of the intangible like that of light, sound, and color and heat. We can see light and color, we can hear sound, and we can feel heat. There is a way to contact spirit too; we must first learn how to do it. Galileo gave us the basics to capture the rhythm of life and the vibration of spirit through the pendulum.

An oscillator is anything that has the ability to hold the rhythm of the earth. How does this rhythm work? It is a combination of polar magnetics, gravity, solar energy and the energy that is created through multiple reactions.

Our bodies are oscillators, just like everything that carries or holds an electro-magnetic current. Some use a pendulum as a tool for divination, asking yes or no questions with the response being a subtle movement in the sway of the pendulum that is determined by the diviner. Tuning forks and dowsing wires work on the same premises of electro-magnetics. I use a pendulum with a diamond as a weight during healing sessions to observe the oscillatory behavior of our biorhythm keepers, the *suprachiasmatic nuclei* that naturally exists within our bodies and control our body's cycles. Pendulum work taps into and amplifies the inner rhythms that drive the very existence of all life within the universe. Cellular and celestial bodies both move and support life due to the electrical pulse and divine nature within every atom. Preparing the body with a polarizing massage, we can move into working on tuning the rhythms that control every aspect of our health drawing balance, clarity, and calm to the mind, body, and spirit. Tuning the seven major chakras by harnessing the natural magnetizing charge of sunlight and aligning each chakra to a harmonizing musical note can help align the rhythms of the body with the rhythms of our Earth and the rhythms that drive the cosmos.

Fourteen

The Importance of Intention

It is important to recognize ourselves as beings capable of both good and bad. It is important to know that we all have a choice to do what is right or what is wrong. We all have different limitations, capabilities, and natural talents. We must choose to understand and accept ourselves first, and to accept that each person we interact with also has a choice and a will, as well as the ability to be very good or very bad. Our character and integrity are the ways that we let the world know what kinds of choices we are making. I have met many revered people, who have so much experience that could be passed down, but they have allowed themselves to become closed, bitter, shallow, or angry. Therefore, their outstanding experience cannot be clearly passed on. We all have our own personal cycles and no matter what our actions are, we can sometimes be derailed. This is when our true intention and passion for what we strive to create from the core of our being comes through. This intention and passion will always show your true character. If we choose to follow our greatest good and best intentions, we have done our best. We must try to stay as clean and clear as possible to perform healing work. Working energetically with the chakras and using tools such as diamonds and other gemstones requires an intention that is very pure. I know many "energy workers," but they are not people I would invest my energy with. All people are like banks. There can be a lot of unknown fees and charges that are hidden at the time of service. These people are messing with stuff that will cause them harm and you harm. Most of the time, it only takes being around them a time or two before their intentions and character become clear.

A healer can have a bad day, be it an argument, an accident, or an illness. However, if they know what they are doing, they can drop these incidents at the door, wash their hands, take a few deep breathes, and move right into their work. It is not that the incidents do not exist;

they do not matter when it comes to helping another person be well. Of course, if a healer never works through their own issues, they will not be clear enough to heal anymore. It would be like saying that I would not jump into the water to save a child from drowning because I am experiencing a sniffle. This is different from someone who has lived with pneumonia for a long time. People can have a spiritual pneumonia and be physically and spiritually incapable of helping another human being.

Humans, by nature feel compassion for all things, and if they can, they will try to help if they feel the pain of a living creature. This empathic emotion becomes dull or deadened if they have too much pain to deal with. Therefore, we must recognize what causes us pain, do what we can to minimize the pain and take the time to heal ourselves, so we have enough to help others if that is what we choose to do. People who work in the field of healing experience so much joy from helping another person that this is why they have chose to make healing a lifestyle. There is plenty to heal within ourselves and this is something we must be doing everyday with intention. There are techniques for healing ourselves, but much of self-healing is individual. As long as we experience joy, laughter, and happiness everyday, we are healing. To encourage healing in other is to experience healing ourselves. To encourage damage and pain in another is to encourage the same within ourselves.

Live with intention. Know that every choice has a consequence that is generally good or bad. This consequence is not separated from the choice, it must always be considered. How we experience or deal with these consequences depict our character and will eventually create our intentions. This is interpreted though integrity and personal constitution. Take responsibility for your actions and much will right itself.

Fifteen

The Magic of Prayer and Manifestation

Silence is the gift of Nature,
Although once you seek silence in Nature
You find beauty,
A trace of everything that ever was.
Trees are not just trees,
They are medicine, shade, and a home for birds alive with song
Air is more than empty space,
It is the catalyst for all we perceive,
An empty slate for the vibration of life.
Bringing pieces of nature into your home
Reminds you to seek beauty
And tempts you to seek silence.

A person who wants to will their intention shall create a safe place that they use to remind themselves of the beauty they keep in their lives. Sometimes an altar can evolve out of it or it may just be a fireplace, or a special place you like in your yard. It can be encouraging to place pictures, found items and given items at this place to help create an area of sanctuary. Many metaphysical stores make a business out of creating sacred space. Utilize them if you need to. The point is to create a place where an individual feels that he or she can touch spirit on whatever level that is possible.

The next step to manifesting and prayer is learning to be still and by yourself. Learning to focus for 10-20 minutes on what one truly wants in their lives. This means turn off your TV, cell phone, and your radio. If you want something, you must familiarize yourself by playing the visual image of succeeding in that goal over and over again in your mind, each step becoming more real and every accomplishment easier to obtain. A person has to want to take time to address what they want to create for themselves; otherwise it is in our nature to want things that other people that are around us want. The media has a way of imposing images of desire and need on the populace. Learning to map the steps we have to take in order to obtain a personal goal can be confusing and this is why so many people take to journaling. The potent magic of a spell is in the intention of its caster. If you can write down in a very detailed manner the way that you would like something to unfold and then sit for a few moments with good intention playing the situation out in your mind, you will find that your energy towards the manifestation becomes very clear and pure. A lot of anxiety and confusion dissipates with each moment of focus spent. The more an individual wants something the more their energy moves in a positive way to create it for themselves. If we simply believe that it is possible to obtain our goals, then we have broken down half of the barriers that keep us from them. If one needs to make a physical reminder of how one wants to manifest a goal, they should write it down and put it somewhere that they look everyday, like a bathroom mirror or an alter. You can use affirming statements like:

> I, _____ wish to manifest what I **want** and **need** in my future. I understand that I have to obtain these goals through intention, will, focus, and purity of purpose. My goals are_____
>
> _____
>
> _____. All of this I manifest for the good of myself and for the good of everyone I encounter.

When people want something, usually they ask for prosperity or wisdom of some kind. There is always a process. If you would like to own a house, but you have no job, you must work on getting a job first. If you want a job, but you have no transportation, you must work on manifesting transportation first. If you do not know how to drive, you must take the responsibility upon yourself to study the driver's manual and pay the fee to take the test successfully. So really, in this case, you cannot manifest a house, before you have a driver's license, and this is exactly how most attempts to manifest go wrong. The only way to accomplish any goal is by knowing, to the extent of your foresight, the steps one must take in the process. You must write down all of the steps that are known to you that are necessary in obtaining your goal. You must sit in silence and focus on one step at a time and see yourself paying your test fee, and then taking the drive, see your license in hand as you step into your vehicle that will take you to your job interview. Look down and notice what kind of clothes you are wearing and how calm you feel. Now walk though the door of your future employer and see yourself successfully doing the job. You must dedicate time to manifest what you want in your life. Otherwise, you will wake up one day, look around, and feel deeply disappointed when nothing you have is what you wanted. Any person who wishes to will something into their lives must work very hard to do so, accepting the length of the process, the steep hills and valleys one goes through to get to the end of the journey. Be patient and persistent and know that if the accomplishment is yours to have, you will have it in time.

It was while I was receiving my training on the island of Maui that I began to recognize the power of prayer and manifestation. Soon after I arrived on the island, I was instructed to leave a prayer and a gift to the Island Goddess Pele. There is an Earth altar set up above a small inlet below the lava field known as the King's Highway, beyond the end of Wailea road. I returned there many times to give thanks for the blessings I received while I lived on the island. The whole island I realized over time is an amazing Earth altar. The strangest things began to happen to me as soon as I arrived on the island. I was able to obtain what I needed and all I had to do was ask for it. The people who helped me to establish myself as a resident, had told me about the magic of the islands and though I thought it all sounded nice and idealistic, it seemed a little too magical to be a reality. Some of it was and some of it was not. I spent a lot of time alone. During this alone time, I taught myself how to visualize and manifest. I learned that it helped to think only progressively towards situations and people. I found that if I wished for a situation to end, it soon would. I found that if I thought angry thoughts about an acquaintance or cursed a friend for doing me wrong, an aspect of the situation would always come back to haunt me. I had to change the negatives that were buried in my character into positives. It took me a great amount of drive, patience, acceptance, and time to change the thinking patterns that did not help me. Still, I work on this every day. I found that my intuition always led me exactly where I needed to be. I learned to trust my passage and not feel so confused and anxious about what the future held. I learned that I could not manipulate another's path for my greater good, as this is a backwards way of thinking. I began to develop my ideas about give and take—positives and negatives. All anyone has to do is choose the situations that appear to be what their soul is deeply yearning for and that which feels natural and righteous.

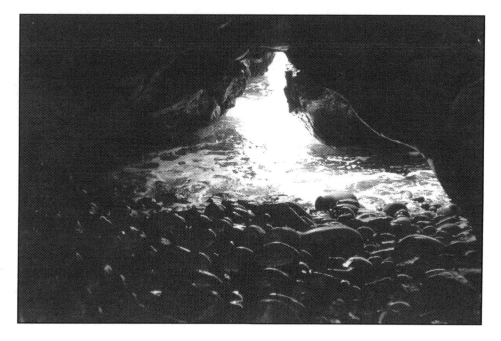

Cave near the Sea

- ℞ Create an altar
- ℞ Make time for silence
- ℞ Keep a journal or write down personal manifestations to keep in your place of manifestation and prayer
- ℞ Focus on visualizing your prayers and manifestations
- ℞ Believe in what you dream

Sixteen

The Workings of Prayer

Many believe that a God that resides in Heaven, the creator of all things, answers a prayer. Cultures that base their spiritual beliefs on the natural world often pray to the gods that control their seasons and the success of their crops, causing desirable weather patterns for the survival of their families and communities. Some choose to be outside where the wind is blowing, at the edge of a pool of water, or amidst the trees in the forest. The most accepted and conventional way of prayer in western societies is performed in a church or temple.

There is a feeling that comes over a person who is close to spirit when they pray. Maybe a warm light or an atmosphere of protection surrounds them. I usually have a feeling that there is always a connection being made with the spirits that are around me and the better will of those people who are around me in my daily life. I try to act right in my world, creating situations that reflect how I want the outcome of each day to be. I take responsibility for what is mine, I let go of situations that affect me in a negative way, and I accept my limits, boundaries, and skills for what they are. When I pray for something, I believe that I am positively influencing the energies or situations involved with the prayer.

Mostly, people need to love what they believe in. Just be happy with whom you are and the things that bring you closer to the divine. If one finds this in their garden, in a Buddhist temple, in the Catholic Church, or taking a hike out in nature with the redwoods, it matters not where you find it. Just find it. One must look into their soul and turn that beauty outward for the world to see. As long as your prayers support the good of all, you are making a positive influence on all of the energy that surrounds you. Prayer is a positive choice. We cannot count on miracles, but if we do all that is in our power to bring forth something for the good of all, chances are that our passion and charisma will affect others around us. This is how one brings about a positive movement. Miracles are only miracles if you do not believe that the change is possible. Keep your integrity, be honest, work hard for the good of all, know your boundaries, and encourage others to follow their dreams. This is the way to choose a positive outcome. This is the working of prayer.

Seventeen

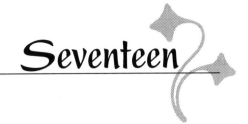

Diamonds

This subject brings this book full circle. Diamonds, mysterious, brilliant, coveted, expensive, and rare, diamonds…

My experience using some of the most extraordinary diamonds in the world as healing tools was the catalyst for this book. The Diamond Information Center brought together a group of people to create diamond treatments for their 2005 Academy Awards DIC event that was held in the third week of February. I was asked if I would be interested in creating a treatment for the event, by my spa director J. Jarnot of The Carneros Inn. I accepted the offer and began studying diamonds immediately. As a practitioner of the healing arts and a student of metaphysics, I was already familiar with all other gemstones and I was very excited to have a reason to add diamonds to my idea tank. What I found out was amazing. At first, there was little to no information on diamonds being used as tools for healing. No information on colored diamonds and their individual healing properties was available. I quickly concluded that I would have to delve deep into color and light therapies and how color and light affect gemstones and rock matter. Trying to identify the areas that seemed relevant in the field of the healing arts to this proposed diamond therapy was the easy part. Light, refraction, rainbow and prismatic color, cuts and faceting, resistance to damage, diamonds in jewelry and the wedding tradition, applying diamonds to the chakras and how I could use them to effect the aura, would all become a part of my finished diamond treatment. The project became overwhelming. In order for the therapy to work, I had to understand the concepts that I would be working with and talking about. I had to formulate my ideas on paper, be able to perform it, and most of all, believe in it. Being a collector of crystals and gemstones, I knew about the calming and balancing effects that these stones have on a person when they are placed around the home. They can be entrancing as well as healing.

The origin of the word diamond goes back to the word adimantum and then to adamant meaning unyielding or impenetrable. Webster's dictionary actually states, "adamant: a legendary stone thought to be impenetrable." In the 16th century, the word diamond had officially evolved into its current use. Adamantine is a diamond. Some diamond-lovers believe them to cure disease, avert calamity, and ward off evil spirits and phantoms. I have also heard that people use them as protective amulets and raw as protectors of crops, homes, and livestock from infestations, disease, natural disasters, and phenomenon, such as lightning. Shamans from many cultures claim them as healing tools and they have been associated with at least one archaeological sight in Africa, where a leather pouch was found having diamond material along with other healing tools.

Diamonds have a strong magnetic charge, especially when light passes through them. They have what scientist call a phosphorescent quality and become electrically (+p) when exposed to UV light. P.J. Fisher writes in *The Science of Gems*, "Many diamonds display a sky blue color called fluorescence, when subjected to ultra-violet radiation. The color is inconsistent and can appear faint to brilliant. It is suggested that this strange property be used as a means of identifying pieces of diamond, like a fingerprinting process. We also know that diamonds act as oscillators or conductors of energy, like quartz crystals used in watches and radios. Diamonds as well as quartz crystals are called piezoelectric material. These materials emit an electrical charge when stressed. When stressed in one plane the material will discharge energy in a plane perpendicular to the plane of stress. This characteristic shows that the forces holding the crystal lattice together are electric as well as molecular and ionic (*Lightseeds*, Wind, W. and Reid, A.; Prentice Hall Press 1988).

This crystal lattice can also be used an amplifier of vibration if fashioned in the right way. Piezoelectric material can act like a timekeeper as well as an amplifier of vibration, relaying information in the form of vibration in a clear manner. The record players of the seventies and eighties were revolutionalized when Stanton, a purveyor of fine audio equipment came out with the diamond stylus. This was a needle used to pick up the delicate vibrations encoded in the vinyl of any record. Diamond tipped needles picked up on the finely encoded dips and chinks that create the vibrations of sound played through the copper wires of the speaker system. Before the diamond stylus, a needle was more like a nail or a piece of wire. Over time, these archaic needles would ruin the vinyl by slowly rubbing down the dips and chinks, making the sound of the record hazed and scratchy. It seems clear to me that these stones can hold an oscillating vibration, clearly relay vibrational energy, in particular sound, and become magnetically charged through the ways of sunlight! These properties seem like natural characteristics for a stone as revered as the diamond. The nature of this gemstone became more alluring and dynamic with each reference I discovered.

Diamonds are fine in their atomic structure, making them very clear allowing for extraordinary luster, fire, and refraction. A diamond's chemical composition has a specific order that gives them the color and fire that makes them so very desirable to the consumer. The amount of light rays that are bent by the diamond along with its luster or the amount of light reflected from its surface determines the refractive index or RI of the diamond. The gemstone's birefringence is the difference between its minimum and maximum RI. Each facet of a diamond increases its fire and luster, each cut acting like a mirror helping to reflect the light as it passes through.

Diamonds are the hardest natural material that we know of, but not the toughest. Cleavage, cracks, and pores are the elements that predict a stones resistance and hardness. High quality diamonds used in jewelry have the least amount of cleavage and blemish. This allows for a lot of the lower quality material to be utilized for industrial demands, mostly in heavy-duty cutting machinery. The diamond has a weaker atomic structure and when mixed with a cleavage line and considerable force from another hard substance, the diamond can fracture. Therefore, despite their hard nature, they are not the toughest stone. In fact, Jadeite is the toughest stone. Hero of Alexandria points out that the pores of a diamond are too small to create the vacuum effect that normally causes a stone to combust and fracture under exposure to fire. This makes them almost incombustible.

The premise of this treatment is that I am using an oscillator or a natural timekeeper of the earth, the diamond, to tune the suprachiasmatic nuclei or SCN, the controlling oscillator of our bodies. By doing this I hope to create a reaction of cyclical balance. It takes recognizing the role of many elements to make a connection. All I am doing is utilizing the information that I have learned along the way. We all know by now that the third eye is the sixth chakra and the home of the suprachiasmatic nuclei, which is located within the hypothalamus, the regulator of the endocrine system, hormones, and their glands. Among other things, the hypothalamus houses the pineal gland. The optic nerve connects to the hypothalamus making its influence on the body through our perception of light and color or the lack of it. Intuition and the way we perceive others in a spiritual way are all aspects attributed to the third eye. All of the chakras connect to the minor circadians, found within clumps of nervous tissue and are offshoots of the main SCN in the hypothalamus. It appears that we make the greatest impression on the sixth chakra, but it is necessary to create balance in all of them in order to create a lasting affect.

While creating the treatment I concluded that our Chromalive light pen worked very well with the super-clear diamonds. The less blemishes the diamond had, the purer the magnetized energy it produced. I use gemstones and in particular diamonds to create a miniature atmo-sphere of magnetic energy. As I pass the light through the stone, instantly charging it with a positive electrical charge and increasing its magnetism, I set the stone on fire with light and color created by a prismatic reaction. Color is produced when light passes through the gem-stone. A natural property of gemstones is their ability to break white light up into the separate waves that are the seven colors of the rainbow spectrum. Wherever this light reflects, moves, and touches, it affects the area, because light alone creates a charge. This charge affects the molecules surrounding the gemstone. Since we are placing these gemstones on the body in the area of the chakras, we can assume that the magnetic charge is affecting the chakras, their color, the corresponding bodily systems, and the general area they are placed. Because the eye catches what color is not absorbed by the surface of a gemstone, this must mean that the diamonds surface absorbs none of the colors, therefore reflecting all of them. The eye recognizes all of the seven colors in the rainbow spectrum when looking at a diamond. This stone absorbs nothing and reflects everything intensely. This is not the case with many semi-precious gems, making a diamond different, rare, and a privilege to work with as a tool for healing.

The pineal gland receives and responds to sensory information from the optic nerves; it is sometimes referred to as the third eye. Optically, we are affected by everything that surrounds us. The pineal gland uses information regarding changing light levels to adjust its output of melatonin; melatonin levels increase during the night and decrease during the day. This cyclic variation is an important time keeping mechanism for the body's internal clock and the bodies sleep cycles (*The human body in health and disease*, 2nd ed., Thibodeau/Patton, Mosby press 1997).

The positive reaction of applying light and color to diamonds and other gemstones, and a magnetic charge to the chakras and the body is in the way that our bodies react to their in-fluence. It is probable that over-exposure to any of them can create imbalances. The amount that we expose people to these influences in a healing setting is never applied in the extreme. Color can improve and influence the mood in a positive way, as well as providing the type of energy that helps to tune the SCN, repair the aura and therefore encouraging balance within the systems of the body. UV light or natural sunlight encourages the production of vitamin d and is scientifically proven to help regulate the cyclical nature of the glands of the endocrine system, which provides homeostasis and over-all health to human beings. Gemstones are visual beauties adding to the manifestation of health by providing a focal point and a unique molec-ular structure that determines the way light and color are perceived by the body and continues to produce fascination in all those who admire them. Magnetics play a central role in the functioning of everything that functions in the world. From the natural orbit of the Earth to the way a child goes down a slide, magnetism and the laws of gravity help us to understand the way each cell in the world affects the next one. Positives and negatives play a role in everything I can think of. People write plays about it, form theories on it, create religious and spiritual practice out of it, and live by the rules of the opposition of positive and negative. The positives and negatives in this life control the flow of all things.

Eighteen

Jewelry as Medicine

Obviously, if the reader has made it this far into the book, he or she believes in the power and uses for gemstones and crystals as healing tools. Whether you wear a stone because it is your birthstone, you have exchanged vows, it is an inherited item, or you just could not resist making it a part of your collection, stones are valuable to you for one reason or another. My experience with this highly prized stone, the diamond, began when I was asked to create healing treatments using them. Originally, my information was based on their color and the qualities already known about diamonds. The information presented below is revised and revisited based on my current experience with the stones as tools for healing.

Colorless or Clear Diamond: (Crown) Ultimately promotes innocence and purity in chastity and spirit. Acts like a window to the soul allowing for the true immaculate nature of the person who wears it. Allows openness to spiritual realms by allowing for support and communication between the wearer and the personal spirituality that the wearer believes in. Provides revelations to the keeper through ways of spiritual and universal truths. A master healer. An oscillator and natural timekeeper. Diamond is one of the piezoelectric stones holding an electrical charge when placed under pressure. A diamond becomes magnetized as soon as UV light shines though it and enables the diamond to be activated for healing. Can be used at any chakra. It is a purifier of all energies.

When using the diamond in a pendulum—one wants to be directly in the sunlight or able to use a portable UV light. Casting the prism or light through the diamond and onto the client is great visually, but it is also tuning the space in the aura that it reaches. The diamond does this by filling the bio-field and covering the body with powerful refracted light, helping to regulate the natural rhythm of the physical body, especially the endocrine system and the nervous system. UV light can magnetize anything that it touches, but the diamond is an easy and quick tool to magnetize. It is a great tool for tuning and divination at the third eye chakra.

When exchanging wedding rings, the couple wants to keep the rings tied together and in a silk bag filled with herbs of protection, love, and sacredness. These rings should be kept on an altar with a candle burning for many days. One should also place the vows in the candlelight so that the words are illuminated and made pure. One should pray and write out blessings that the owner wants to associate with the rings and the union. Sacred items of love, like a picture, a poem, and tokens of love can all be placed on the altar in honor of couple being united. Consciously lying out what matters, what is meaningful, and what has brought you to this point in your lives. On the day of ceremony, the rings should be untied and dropped into a bowl of living water to symbolize the great union of two souls.

The diamond has historically always been a stone of great power, the clearest and mostly flawless always being reserved for royalty. I believe it had an effect on the wearer that can be used to boost the self-esteem and for self-promotion. Diamonds creates a feeling of grace and beauty in the wearer. These stones have the ability to affect the chakras in a localized way and extend its cast of fire and luminescence to the biofield and the subtle energy of color or the lack of it in places in the bio-field, which reflect the balances and imbalances of the physical body. Has an over-all energizing and healing effect on the physical body and its bio-field.

Purple/lavender diamonds: (Third Eye) Mysticism and psychic phenomenon surround this stone making it useful at the third eye chakra. Being a stone of transformation, it should be used or worn during prayer, channeling, manifestation, and ceremonies performed with positive intention. The lavender diamond brings insight though the dreamtime and encourages meditation and mediation. I had a client go into an out of body experience while I used this stone at the third chakra, so be prepared to hold a grounded space for your client to do their work. The third eye chakra is easily affected, so this stone should always be cleaned well before it is used for energy work. This stone allows people to tap the universal mind. The lavender diamond assists the wearer in the search for spiritual attainment. Trust hunches and instincts while wearing this stone.

Blue diamonds: (Throat) The blue diamond is an amazing stone. It is a stone for writers, artists, musicians, and performers of spoken word, actors, and all people who depend on their abilities of communication for their livelihood. It is a strong stone that brings muddled thoughts into a clear verbal form. It slows cellular movement and allows for healing to occur. The blue diamond promotes the stability of healthy cells during disease. Encourages sleep and allows for a quieting of the brain, helping to stop the surge of racing thoughts. Allows the wearer to slow down and take the time to enjoy simple pleasures like staring at the ocean or smelling the flowers, realigning one with nature. Use at the throat chakra.

Pink diamonds: (Heart) This is a stone of the heart, you will know as soon as you touch it. This stone helps those struggling to gain compassion for humanity. It allows its keeper to identify faults within humanity and themselves, allowing for forgiveness and for shortcomings. Spreading the radiance of a pink diamond over the heart chakra allows for the healing of emotional wounds going back to birth. This stone should be great for people who have lost their parents through adoption or death. Acceptance and forgiveness is key with this stone. Those who have loved ones who are away at way can find comfort by wearing this stone. The practitioner who uses this stone should be in a state of emotional balance before they lay it on another person, because it strongly creates release in the heart chakra. Your client is likely to have an emotional release if the time is right for them. It has qualities similar to an opal. The pink diamond is a stone for those who grieve, as well as humanitarians, healers, group leaders, and counselors.

Green diamonds: (Heart) The green diamond comes in many shades and is a gift to us from the earth. This stone is meant to be worn and used for healing. Healing physical ailments and wounds that start with the heart, it allows for real balance in the physical body. It allows the body to rejuvenate through relaxation or rest. The green diamond reflects the slow rejuvenation and self-care that is naturally apart of the Earth's cycle. Can cause an upheaval in the heart, causing what seems like disaster, yet revealing what is righteous and healthy for the wearer. Connects directly to the muscle memory and can help in the healing of emotional, mental, and physical abuse and distress. A great stone for body workers. Constantly reminding us of the natural cyclical action of breakdown and decay followed by re-birth. Is likened to the season of spring.

Yellow diamonds: (Solar Plexus) This stone symbolizes the kind of connection held between the child and the mother. It has a pure energy of nurturing and love. It can be passed between friends, family, and lovers. It is a very healing stone that works on the breath and the diaphragm. The way we bring in our breath and how much we allow ourselves to experience and enjoy life is brought to light when wearing this stone. A yellow diamond can balance the pancreas, glandular and lymphatic systems. It relates to the sweetness of life and can help us break out of hibernation or out of the shell we have used to protect our emotional selves and what we see as vulnerable within our physical and spiritual selves. Allow JOY! Allow opening. Allow love, camaraderie and partnership.

Orange diamonds: (Sacral) Orange is alive, just look at it! This stone is connected to the lower organs of the digestive tract and the sexual organs. It vibrates closely to the Sun's natural light, enlivening the wearer with solar like energy. Orange diamonds stimulate tissue regeneration. Deep desires can be brought to the surface along with long desired manifestations concerning the physical body. Brings joy and cheer to the wearer. A vivacious stone that helps people to live out-loud. Promotes self-esteem, personal power, and attracts success. A great stone to wear to an interview or an important date. Encourages creativity, spontaneity, and self-promotion. Orange diamonds can also act as a protective force for a woman who is carrying a child.

Red diamonds: (Root) This color is the most rare to have. The red diamond that I worked with was just over a carat and was worth over a million dollars. It is powerful at the root chakra, representing the movements of spirit below and above. This stone has a way of connecting the wearer to both heaven and earth. This stone helps to connect us to the deep churning and movements of magma, the life giving substance of the earth, once dry the magma acts as a magnetic force within our Earth. In this way, it helps to draw to you what you feel very passionate or strongly towards. Diamonds are 3/4$^{th's}$ as old as the earth and act as record keepers. This make the red diamond a perfect heirloom piece. The red diamond allows you to feel proud of where, who, and what you have come from, allowing the wearer to feel at ease with their past, especially in love. This stone reflects your will to live and holds an imprint of the passion and drive one has in this life to survive.

Brown diamonds: (Root) Encourages the wearer to work through the seasons of the emotions with grace, seeing the beauty in transformation, rather than focusing on the growing pains. This stone symbolizes the breath, the ebb and flow of taking in and letting go. Deeply connected to the earth, this stone helps to ground its keeper and aids in finding the peace that accompanies meditation. This stone is perfect for someone who feels directly connected to the trees, flowers, mountains, lakes, and rivers. It is a romantic stone, reminding us of our ancestors and of the generations past. This is an appropriate stone to wear when one is out on the town or in a large group as it encourages clear thoughts and allows the wearer to break from the crowd while still being in it. The phrase, "be in the world, but not of it," is an appropriate phrase here. Protecting one from the materialistic and those that are only concerned with surface issues.

Black diamonds: (Root) A black diamond can absorb infinite amounts of negative energy, and allows the wearer to transcend sadness and vulnerability, moving forward in the higher goals of homeostasis. The black diamond represents the opposite opportunity for light transference as a clear diamond. It absorbs any energy that is trapped with you that needs to be released. This stone allows one to move forward by encouraging the wearer to open what has been closed by casting light in the darkness and allowing the wearer to bring their secrets or mistakes to the table. Much like, 'letting your skeletons out of the closet'. It is a good stone to have when someone passes away or after a break-up. It connects us to earthly things and the evolution of the universe. It is a stone used as a scrying or fortune telling tool.

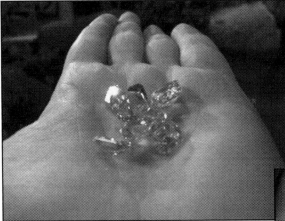

Hand full of Colored Diamonds (42 Carats)

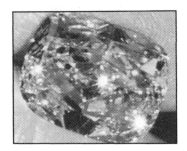

Colorless and Flawless

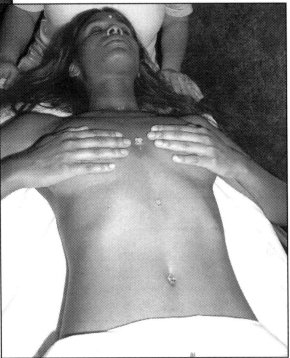

Joy Bryant with Diamonds on Chakras

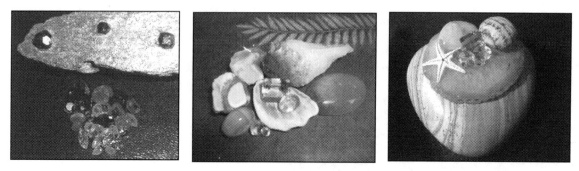

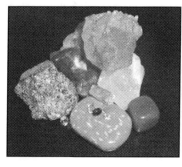

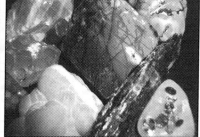

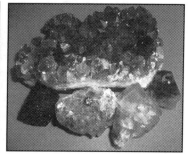

Red Colored Stones   Orange Colored Stones   Yellow
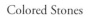
Colored Stones

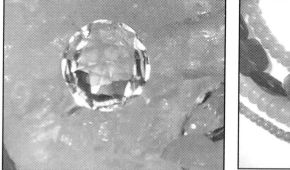

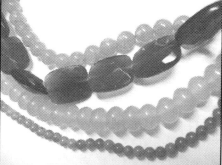

Green Colored Stones   Blue Colored Stones   Purple
Colored Stones

Clear or White Colored Stones   Strands of Color

The following is a short list of my favorite gemstones that I enjoy using for healing outside of diamonds. If you already own any of them, perhaps you know how special they are. These descriptions will help you to understand how they can help you use them as aids for self-healing or guided healing. Placed around the home or used for jewelry these are some of the most amazing stones! Much of what I have learned comes from carrying around Melody's book *Love is in the Earth*. I feel she has done a great job of compiling information and considering many sources. She holds degrees in mathematics and science and is a representative known around the world for her detail and love on the subject of crystals and gemstones. This book is a bible for those who collect crystals and gemstones. I would like to give thanks at this time for Melody's work, without it I simply would have to study a lifetime to compile this type of vast and definitive knowledge.

Obsidian: (Root) This stone acts like a shield against negativity, transforming negative vibrations within the environment. It helps to dissipate anger, anxiety, fear, and sadness. It is protective and keeps the holder out of harms way. Obsidian should be kept in the pocket of those who are in a time of transition and vulnerable to outside influences. This is a perfect stone for someone who is experiencing deep loss or grief. It is a very sharp stone and caution should be taken in handling it if it has any sharp edges. It acts like a black hole, sucking in negative emotions and energies, absorbing it and letting it go back to the earth to be recycled into new clean energy. Obsidian should be placed all over the house, especially under the bed and around the room one sleeps in most.

Red Ruby: (Root) An excellent shielding stone against psychic attack. It is said to protect the carrier from unhappiness, distressing dreams, and lightning. The ruby encourages the wearer to follow bliss. It can conquer darkness on all levels. A ruby can be used to promote a healthy blood flow. This is a great stone for someone who is pregnant. It can help in the optimum formation of the Children in the embryonic state. It is excellent for re-birthing and for releasing blockages that restrain one from the spiritual path. It has been used as a rod–like conductor of atmospheric electricity, providing a pathway to the Earth and to the user, for electrical and magnetic forces. This is a stone of passion that reflects the individual's stamina for survival and their will to live. The ruby is associated with the mythical bird, the phoenix.

Carnelian: (Sacral Chakra) Helps in the treatment of neuralgia, gallstones, Kidney stones, pollen allergies, and colds. This stone provides safety to the wearer from catastrophe. Helps the wearer to feel safe and promotes trust. Carnelian promotes analytical thought and rational thinking. A deep churning of life can be stirred while wearing carnelian. This is a stone of vitality and exudes the vibration of true adventure and exploration. Wear while traveling far away from home.

Peach/Orange Calcite: (Sacral Chakra) Calcite is an oscillator when placed under pressure and an energy amplifier. It brings forth a polarized prismatic energy, which engenders a spectrum of energy to clear and to activate all of the chakras. Placing an orange calcite at the sacral plexus will clear and activate the chakra and provides a sweeping action that clears the remaining centers. This stone works ridding the kidneys, pancreas, and spleen of dis-ease and imbalances.

Citrine: (Solar Plexus) Citrine like Kyanite does not absorb or retain any negative energy. These are the only two stones of this kind. Helps to acquire and keep wealth. It activates, opens, and energizes the solar plexus by directing personal power , creativity, and energy needed to enhance the physical body. Helps one to laugh without restraint. Diminishes "muddy" areas in the aura and physical body. Relates heavily to the intellect. Has been used to fight degenerative diseases. Should be used as a filter at the solar plexus to allow only the positive energy associated with gold/yellow.

Green Tourmaline: (HEART) Helps the wearer to see with the heart as it opens the throat chakra. Tourmaline helps to bring compassion to the keeper in the form of male energy. Love can be had without attachment. Encourages the powerful healing energy found by using herbs or eating fresh garden vegetables and fruits. Transforms negative energy into positive energy. This stone helps to regenerate the heart, thymus, ductless glands, and the immune system. Tourmaline balances the energy meridians of the body. This stone is likened to the sea, illuminating light from within and without. Holding a deep knowledge of all things natural and ancient, tourmaline will work its way right into the soul of its keeper.

Turquoise: (Throat) Tibetan shamans use it for its protective and spiritual properties. It brings all energies to a higher level. It brings communication skills to emotional issues, creativity, and intuition, while allowing for compassion. It is said to protect its holder from environmental pollutants. Turquoise assists thoughtful oral and written communication. This stone produces a polarization effect to the physical and subtle bodies. This is a stone with a deep earthy quality that aids in keeping one connected to themselves during outdoor meditation. A great stone for people who enjoy chanting and singing.

Sapphire: (Throat) Sapphires assist in communication. They brings a depth of beauty of thought over the user. It is known as the stone of prosperity, sustaining the gifts of life. This stone brings the focus of energy to the cellular levels. It strengthens the walls of the veins. A sapphire can help to purify trapped energy caused by holding your tongue and not being able to speak your truth. This stone encourages clear interaction with the people around the wearer. It is used in shamanic practices for clearing atmospheric energy.

Kyanite: (Third Eye) Melody says this stone never needs clearing or cleaning, but I suggest dipping it in a river or glacial water. It does not accumulate negative energy. It makes an excellent stone for chakra work. Kyanite aligns the chakras automatically and immediately. It is a perfect atone to use in a pendulum. It is a stone that should be worn by those who are doing travel around water. Kyanite encourages protection while swimming. Connects to the sky and the cosmos and has an elemental feeling of air. Kyanite provides access to information through the dream-state. This stone support conscious connections between the higher levels of the intuition and the heart. It dispels confusing spiritual issues.

Amethyst: (Third Eye) This is a stone that is connected to the intellect and the influence of the divine. Amethyst promotes the transfer of information to the wearer from the cosmic source. This stone protects the wearer from nightmares and spiritual possessions. The stone represents contentment in spirituality. It assists in the assimilation of new ideas. It has, in current and ancient times been used to support sobriety. It is a great stone for someone who is looking to change an addictive personality. It helps stabilize mental disorders and provides relief from insomnia. Amethyst stimulates the sympathetic nervous system and the endocrine system to work in precise performance. Amethyst allows one to realize the divine nature within themselves and helps one to accept their individual role in the grand structure of the universe.

Quartz: (Crown Chakra) This is the first stone that one should experiment with on a metaphysical level. Quartz has both a piezoelectric quality as well as a pyroelectric quality; meaning the polarity of the quartz crystal changes when it is either subjected to pressure or held in your hand. The tip usually being positive and receiving energy until activated, making the tip negative, thus able to emit energy from the tip. These properties make it a great amplifier and transformer for energy. It transfers thought into sound, producing the vibration associated with thought and affecting the environment with the discharged energy. Using this stone can enhance all of the psychic abilities. Quartz induces amplification of the energy field in the location in which it is placed. The Quartz crystal can produce a field of negative healing ions while clearing the surrounding effects of positive ions. It can also counteract radioactivity and radiation.

Opal: (Crown Chakra) It allows clear, true, and spontaneous action. It can be used to assist one in being unseen or invisible. This stone holds a mystic quality and allows people to follow their visions. This is a sacred stone and was used during the Native American Indian vision quest. The opal has a quality of fire that helps it to reflect an amazing amount of color. This makes it a great stone of equality, helping people to feel accepted while helping prejudices to slip away. It can be used as a tool to connect two people together in the dreamtime. Opals help people feel positive and forward moving. Opals hold an imprint of the spirit of an emotion, event, place, or person. I have heard that an opal is fossilized water. This is a stone of magic that can be instantly charged by placing it in a cup of water.

Nineteen

Cleaning Diamonds and other Gemstones

A few elements are essential for energetically cleaning your gems. Living water, sunlight or an open flame, sea salts and a blessing or song help to neutralize all energy.

Living water means water that flows from a natural source over rocks and by trees and is not stagnant in any way. Bottled water does not do the trick. Find a river, lake, spring, creek, or ocean to do this work. It is always important to find a quiet space where one can be alone to focus on the words and energy they need to neutralize their stones. Natural hot springs are a gift from the Earth for cleansing our bodies and our crystals and gemstones.

Sunlight helps to cleanse away bacteria as well as energetically charges a stone by raising the atomic vibration in a stone through pure clean UV light. Light over time turns to thermal energy and thermal energy helps to eradicate anything that does not vibrate to the core molecular structure of the gemstone. One way of using sunlight is to place your stones in a bowl of living water and allow them to sit together undisturbed for a day or two. If you are not near living water, you can use any water with an addition of Celtic or Dead Sea salts to help ionize the water and then leave them out in the sunlight.

There is a difference between candlelight and sunlight. It is a combination of the heat, the light and the smoke that a candle emits that helps to cleanse a stone, not just the light. There are also different reasons to use different mediums of cleansing although sometimes you use what is available at the time. Sunlight is used to cleanse a bulk amount of stones that one may use to do healing work and to place around their home in a way that charges your home with their essence or atomic radiation. Many people do not understand the act of smudging. It is that it is more than it appears. We know that people have been using smoke for centuries

71

to cleanse people spiritually and there is a good explanation for it. While discovering the significance of biological rhythms and the correspondence of the chakra systems, I had an *aha!* moment when I read an insert about smoke and how it stops the natural biorhythms that exist in every living cell as soon as the cells becomes saturated in the smoke. Roger G. Newton recorded this information in his book, *Galileo's Pendulum*. This makes a lot of sense, because one of the most powerful uses for smudging is in clearing humans, land and living space, animals, and tools for healing. Smoke stops the weaker biorhythms left in trace amounts by other humans, animals, bacteria and other residual energies left behind just by living. This allows for a place or object to be cleared of the physical energy that had been associated with it before it was in your possession. The smoke is naturally resinous and adheres to the unwanted molecules carrying them up and away, redispersing them within our atmosphere. Therefore, the key to using candlelight or any kind of smudge tool is an open window or door or a fireplace where the smoke is released. American Indians have used the smoke of sage, cedar, sweet grass, etc., to release energy though the letting of smoke and in blessing land and other items. Many people believe that smoke carries with it the prayers from this world to the next, allowing one to communicate with their ancestors and other influential spirits.

Seawater carries all the minerals and trace elements essential to creating life on our planet. It is important that we know that sea salt absorbs at the same time ironically charges whatever is submerged in it. This means that cleaning your gemstones in real sea salt is much like letting the ocean gently carry away unwanted energy while allowing an ionic charge to take place. William Wilks proposes that one can extract X-rays from ones bones using angle-wires, sea salt, baking soda and the magnetics that already exist in the earth. People that are interested in this should read, *The Science of a Witch's Brew*, by William Wilks. I propose your crystals may be cleaned and re-charged in the same way. I am finding that there is a very specific formula to doing things in a conducive way and with intent towards true purpose and order. Most people do not take time to form true intent and this is why their energy is powerless, not because they "do" or "do not" have it within them.

It is known that burying raw crystals and gemstones in sea salt or sand for up to a year can help to completely erase any connection that it might have with its previous owner. This process is also known to remove oxidization from the physical form of crystals. You may dig a hole in the ground and line it with straw, banana leaves, or any kind of natural fiber. The hole only needs to be 12" to 14" wide by 12" to 14" deep. Place the stones you want to clear and clean into a satchel of natural fibers. Fill the hole with 8 cups full of sea salt, pat flat, place the satchel of stones in the center of the salt, and cover them with another 8 cups of salt. Place more of the natural fibers on top of the salt to seal it in and cover the salt with loose and slightly moist dirt so that it packs tightly. You may leave your stones buried for as long as you want, but I believe that three months to a year is plenty of time. Now your crystals and gemstones are energetically cleared from their previous place or keeper and can be placed around your house, used for healing, given away, or worn again with ease.

Twenty

Programming your Jewelry to Work for you

Once you have cleaned your diamonds or gemstones, you can program each one to be used as a different kind of tool for healing. It is best to buy a nice informative book on the properties of crystals, minerals, and gemstones. The programmer must be prepared to program each crystal based upon its natural properties or qualities. This is based on the shape, size, color, and composition of the stone. For example, you can program an orange diamond for grounding, but it would be more powerful and far more useful if it were programmed for joy, cheer, or charisma. Opals are known to carry with them the emotions of its previous keeper, so clear them well and use water and sea salt, do not ever bury the opal, as they are most likely to become brittle and crack. Once they are clear an opal should be used to signify freedom, diversity, community, and balance of the emotional self. Many books on the market will have comparable descriptions on the properties of the most common gemstones.

Once you have identified the pieces of jewelry that you would like to program, gather a piece of new clean paper, which has not been dyed, bleached, or lined. Natural watercolor paper works well. Next, you must rip off a piece as big as you need and lay it down flat on the table. Next, take a colored pencil that most closely corresponds with the color of your stone and write on the paper how you would like to charge the piece of jewelry or crystal. The person programming the jewelry shall wrap the paper around the jewelry and press the edges into the paper making an imprint, using your fingertips. This is a way of manifesting. Now place this wrapped piece of jewelry in a window to receive UV light, thus magnetizing it with only your prayer wrapped around it.

It is important to write down the way in which you choose to program your pieces of jewelry. This is a very powerful way of manifesting, because you must visualize with direct intent on the exact way you want the talisman or crystal to work for you, going over it in your mind until it is perfectly clear. This may be one of the oldest and most simple ways of casting a spell.

You may take a silk baggie and place the piece inside with the prayer and sleep on it, taking note to the dreams you have, recording them, and looking for clues to see if there is a more specific use for your item. You may also light a candle, passing the piece over the flame and saying many times how you wish to will your intention—leaving the piece in the flickering light of the candle until the candle burns out. Use your best judgment in safety of course.

If this is a piece of jewelry is a family heirloom, you may wish to simply take the piece to a place of flowing water. Holding the piece of jewelry in your hands securely, ask the water to neutralize any energies that belong with the piece, therefore clearing it for you to wear in respect of those who came before you and in connection to the sacred knowledge that is held in your family line and meant to be passed to you.

To stay in touch with someone during your dreamtime, you must clear a stone or piece of jewelry and have them sleep with it under their pillow for a while and then have them give it back to you. Clearing it first and having them sleep with it helps to minimize an influence of other energies on it. The silk satchel creates an atmosphere of natural neutralization, allowing it to be more or less protected from influencing you or charging it with your energy. Be sure to put the item back in its satchel, if you are feeling out-of-sorts or have been in a negative setting, like a seething tavern, etc. You may keep this on an altar in the same room where you sleep or meditate, or you can take the stone out of the silk satchel it came in and put it under your pillow or by your bed.

Twenty One

Gems in History

No one used to facet or modify diamonds or gemstones of any kind. The true essence of a stone was held in the original untouched form. East Indian lore forbid modifying a stone into gem form, convinced that this process might bring about unforetold consequences. Vajra, meaning thunderbolt, was the first documented word used to describe a diamond. Perhaps these folks understood the potential of energy locked within these jewels. According to the American Museum of Natural History, there is archaeological evidence that supports the use and admiration of diamonds and other gemstones dating as far back as 320 BCE. It seems to me that the most reliable evidence always comes out of India with the earliest descriptions found in the 4th century BCE. The chakras were first written about in a Sanskrit manuscript, and later translated by a minister by the name of Kantiliya of the Mauryan Dynasty. As far as archaeological sites go, the only evidence found of diamonds being used as charms in jewelry is in Sri Lanka, India, Thailand, Yemen, and Egypt. The evidence is found in beaded jewelry. Like empty graves, the diamonds have all been picked out of their settings or lost over time. Like a fossil, these beads show what is known as the specific imprint of the first diamond hand drills, a concentric groove. The drill had a thick resinous substance rubbed over a wood or stone conical tip. Diamond chips were rolled into this resin until the tip was covered with the near dust-like diamond material. The tool was hand held and used much like the ancient pestle, but smaller, easier to use and with the purpose of detail. These tools were used for carving, making rough facets, engraving, and drilling. This information is confirmed in China, according to Astronumi.com. Apparently, diamonds were used strictly as an engraving tool being applied to jade and pearls. Yet, archaeological evidence concludes that diamonds were also used 6000 years ago to grind and polish ceremonial stone axes in China (*the Curious Lore of Precious Stones* pg. 289-301).

Perhaps, the industrial benefits were just as important as the spiritual. The Chinese were not the only people who used diamonds as tools for engraving. Diamonds made their way to Rome around 100 CE and Pliny the Elder, of Rome, writes about diamonds being used to engrave sapphires, but also used as talismanic rings. In 23-79 CE, Pliny writes about diamonds in an encyclopedia, "Historia Naturalis", "The substance that possesses the greatest value, not only among precious stones, but among all human possessions is adamas... If one was to test these stones with an anvil, they will resist a blow to such an extent as to make the iron rebound and splitting the anvil."

"Ratnapariksa," of the Buddha Bhatta, is an ancient text written on gems in the 6th century. The natural uncut form of the diamond was very revered at this time and place in history, as well. It explains, "...he having pure body, always carries a diamond with sharp points, without blemish and free from all faults...he will bear happiness, prosperity, children, riches, cows, he will be free from famine, evil spirits, thieves, poison, etc."

In some ways, diamonds became a Buddhist symbol of spiritual virtue. This is displayed by the allowance of different casts of the populace being restricted in wearing only certain colors of diamonds. Obviously, different colored diamonds have always had different values and qualities associated with them. The highest class being priests and rulers or Brahmin, carried the white and colorless diamonds. Their clarity was symbolic of the clarity of their spirit and their minds. Flawless and colorless diamonds have always been the most revered and rare through out history. The Kshatriya or warriors and owners of vast amounts of land were given and allowed to wear diamonds that were red to brown in color. I find it interesting that red diamonds were given to the warrior class, as today these stones are considered one of the rarest and certainly one of the priciest. They were probably awarded these stones to symbolize the blood shed during battle as well as their passion and loyalty to their land. The merchant class or Vaisya wore only the yellow diamond and the Sudra or lower class wore stones that were gray to black in coloration.

Recorded use of diamonds as jewelry or in any form seems to disappear from history about 1000 years after the initial rise of Christianity. This can be associated with the Roman use of diamonds as talismans and the East widely using them as magical charms setting the grounds for Christianity to deem them evil and blasphemous. It appears that the natural trade route went from India through Ethiopia into Alexandria then to Rome and Constantinople. The route made a natural circuit. At around the same time that Christianity was in the height of its manifest the Middle East put a block in the trade route through mass interest in the magical stone. In the 13th century, small amounts of diamonds began appearing for trade and in jewelry. Although diamond rings date back to the 1ˢᵗ and 2ⁿᵈ centuries, the custom became Christianized by the 4ᵗʰ century and this is when the first royal diamond ring to be exchanged during matrimony appeared between Maximilian and Mary the Duchess of Burgundy.

Saint Louis the IX of France (1214-70) found the diamond to be so alluring and tran-cematic that he made a law reserving ownership of all diamonds to the King. Obviously, this was the only way this Saint knew how to keep control over the mysterious lure of a diamond. Knowing of the troubled hearts of men and seeing the envy and jealousy in the eyes of those lucky enough to behold such a stone, he banished them from the eyes and hands of the average person. The dark age of diamonds ended in France in the 17ᵗʰ century when diamonds became prominent in the royal jewelry of both men and women.

The pattern through history is that this gem of amazing brilliance and beauty has always been reserved for leaders of religion and land. Flawless and uncut they symbolized the natural beauty of mind and spirit within the owner. These stones seem to have an unknown power over the people who are trying to obtain them. Christianity, in its height did not approve of the stone being worn or used as talismans or jewelry, as these sorts of adornments could only be seen as aids in working with a power outside that of the Christian God. It is a shame that the main religion of the western world could not see the diamond for what it was, as the people in the East did. I believe that God is in everything, especially a diamond. Few things have held one's glance for as long as the mysterious fire of adamas. Diamonds have had a place on our Earth longer than humans or dinosaurs and the stones will outlast their keepers for as long as the Earth keeps spinning.

*Many references in this chapter are from the Museum of Natural Histories web-site on diamonds.

Twenty Two

Guided Visualization and the Importance of Focus

There is so much going on in our daily lives that it is fair to say that most people do not get to spend enough healthy time with themselves. How often do you hear someone say that they were thinking about the health of their liver, or their little toe, or their pelvis? Mostly, we distract ourselves with the needs of those around us, like our mates, our children, our ailing family members, and mostly our jobs. If you are ailing and need attention and help to reach balance, do you have anyone to count on, beside yourself? Some lucky people can say yes, but for most of us, we are the only ones in charge of our health and our boundaries.

The real point of visualization is making a connection. Most people are in denial about the responsibility we have to ourselves. It is no one's job, but our own, to take care of the quality of life we have. This means how we breathe, how we exercise, how we work, and how we heal. Practicing visualizations for health is a great way to bring calm and relaxation into your day. It can enhance and help create focus in our bodywork treatments, as well. It is important to have a general understanding of the anatomy for deeper visualizations. One should stretch out or be in a comfortable open position, because it is easier to focus. Music should be instrumental or not at all during this time, because song can become very visual and distracting.

ᕒᕱ   Basic visualization for clearing and opening

(use a lemon, grapefruit or orange aroma)

Close your eyes and begin to breathe deeply. Feel the ground that supports you. Know what it feels like to be in your body right now. Know that you are safe and that this is a time for you to unravel and let go. (Let the person breathe for a minute, without any speech). Imagine that with each deep breath that you take in you are pulling in a positive crystal clear energy. This energy sheds light on each cell that it touches. The breath nourishes you more the deeper you breathe in. Every time you breathe out any resinous negative energy that has built up inside of you is being pushed out. Imagine as you take the breath in—the air itself is churning with light filling all of the dark crevices and nooks. As you breathe out--the negative and dark energy stirred up like dust in the sunlight gets blown out of the body with the breath. Each time you finish a breath you can see the tissue in your body glowing pink with vitality until there are no dark crevices left. Keep breathing. Breathe in and hold, breathe out and hold. Repeat.

ᕒᕱ   Visualization for grounding

(use cedar, amber, or frankincense aroma)

Close your eyes and feel the ground around you. Know that you are cradled by the Earth, that she is strong enough to hold you and all that weighs with you. I would like you to imagine that you are laying on soft moss and a bed of leaves in the forest. See the tall strong trees rise around you creating a canopy of green with sparse bits of sunlight that pour through like rays of light after a rainstorm. Know that this is your place. I want you to feel any tension and emotion that you want to let go slip into a puddle at the back of your body. Slowly see this puddle being absorbed by the ground you lay on. Take a few controlled deep breaths letting your whole body relax and sink into the ground just a little bit. Imagine a deep red glow forming in your lower abdomen. As the glow expands, it fills your hips and your pelvis spinning just a bit blasting any blockages or cobwebs out of the area. Now, this red glow pours into your legs like two thick heavy lava flows returning to the earth. The flows reach your knees and it takes a little time, but the lava breaks away any blockages there. Slowly the two flows make it the ankles and the feet—filling the feet like two small pools. Finally, like a dam flooding over, this red lava pours out the soles of your feet like two waterfalls. The lava pours out and down into the earth through cracks and crevices going back to where it came from. You can see the red glow in your abdomen like a bubbling well pouring this thick and heavy fluid down your legs and deep into the earth—pushing through the crust with little effort--connecting you straight to the core of the earth.

ॐ   Visualization for relaxation

(use lavender, vetivert, chamomile, ylang-ylang)

Close your eyes. Begin breathing deeply. Breathe in for ten seconds—breathe out for ten seconds. Notice how your body feels right now. Are you tense, anxious, exhausted, and angry? Just recognize the feeling and decide that for now you are going to make every attempt to let that go. For just a moment, I would like you to imagine what the water looks like when it is calm at sundown. See the water calm and soft, the color of the sky on a reflection of silver or steel. Slowly imagine this water warm and calm flowing in around you lifting you up as if you were as light as a feather, just floating there on the top. Take a few deep breaths. I want you to feel your feet, go ahead, and squeeze them as tight as you can in full flexion and hold for 10 seconds. Release. Feel a tingling sensation and lightness come into your feet. Next, feel your legs, go ahead and tighten them from your calves though your thighs. Hold them as tight as you can for 10 seconds. Release. Feel the sensation of lightness there, too. Now tighten your buttocks and hips as tightly as you can. Hold for ten seconds and release. Notice how light the lower half of your body is. Feel your abdomen, clenching it tight like the biggest sit-up you have ever done and hold for 10 seconds. Release. Feel you spine and all the parts that are connected to it. Arch your back, flex, and hold for 10 seconds. Release. Clinching your fists, squeeze your hands and hold for ten seconds. Release. Flexing your arms only, tense your forearm to your bicep and hold. Take a deep breath and release. Arch your neck back and shrug your shoulders up in flexion. Hold tight to this position for 10 seconds. Release. Lastly, scrunch up your eyes, mouth, and face, push your chin to your chest, and hold for ten seconds. Take three deep breaths and be still. Feel the water holding you still—letting you just float there. Notice how good it feels just to float and be nearly weightless.

Visualization is important because it helps one to identify with their bodies, if they feel pain they understand where it is coming from, if it has a source, and what posture or action has caused the pain to occur. It also gets the client away form the world around them, letting a person just be with themselves and the world you help them to create.

Twenty Three

The Protocols

The following three diamond protocols are an inspired grouping based upon the work that I have performed with the Diamond Information Center. My hope is that one day I will be able to share my work through teaching others who are interested in the healing power held within the diamond. These are the formats I use when working with diamonds and these protocols are very adaptable for use with any kind of crystals or gemstones.

I am providing samples of my personal work, so that you, the reader, can take inspiration in how easy it is to provide this kind of healing to your clients. It is important that anyone who chooses to embark upon this trail of healing feels prepared and called to do so. This is not work for the flighty or the fickle-minded. This work is for the warriors and soldiers of spirit who work on the side of healing and are the caretakers within their worlds. This is not a publicity stunt or meant to fade out like so many fads; this is an ancient art that I believe has been harnessed for centuries by those who could afford the pleasure. This is an era when many of us are able to own our own diamonds and if not a diamond, then very beautiful and powerful crystals and gemstones.

I want to remind the reader that raw diamonds have been the preferred form for Buddhists, Hindis, and many kings, even during times when faceting was available. An untouched and unaltered stone mimics the natural power and brilliance found within and upon our amazing planet.

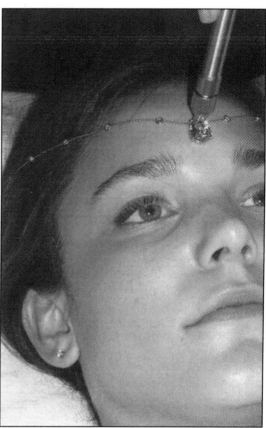

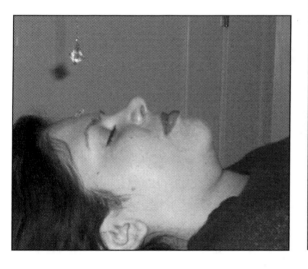

Using a Pendulum to Tune the Chakras

Utilizing UV Light for Healing

Protocol #1

Technical Instruction for Alternative Healing Therapy Using Diamonds

ELEMENTS OF THE THERAPY

A.   1-7 natural or faceted diamonds at .25 minimum carat weight

B.   Pure aromatherapy oil-preferably organic and certified

C.   UV light/solar light in a controllable form and easily utilized by a practitioner of the healing arts

    1.   preferably a light that one can hold or touch to the diamond's surface while in contact with a client

    2.   Example: a UV light pen is suggested to perform diamond therapy accurately, but other appropriate light sources are invited and can be utilized such as solar light therapy bulbs and extended products

D.   An education or extensive experience in the healing arts with a focus on gemstone therapy, chakras and chakra balancing, massage therapy and/or reflexology is required. Along with guided visualization and aromatherapy. This is not a treatment that should be instructed by or taught to anyone who is not pure in his or her intentions towards the facilitation of healing through alternative methods.

DIAMOND AMPLIFICATION AND REFRACTAL THERAPY

Step 1: Introduce the client to the diamonds. Explain why you have chosen the faceted or uncut diamonds for your therapy. Allow the client to touch the diamonds and ask questions.

Step 2: Explain to the client the benefits of using UV light.

Why choose UV light?

UV light is a type of light that is or replicates the Sun's natural energy. UV light provides vitamin D to the human body, which is crucial in the simulation of serotonin and the proper function of the neurotransmitters, which if are not firing correctly will cause imbalances that include depression and insomnia. UV light in particular creates a polar magnetic charge in a diamond. UV light has always been preferred among admirers and professionals to create the prismatic fire exclusive to diamonds.

Step 3: Introduce at least four specialized aromatherapy oils that have been formulated for this treatment. Make sure that the client does not have any allergies that may be triggered by the ingredients in the oils.

Step 4: Ask the client how much they know about their chakras. Feel free to explain that we are utilizing color as a vibration that affects mood, corresponds to the chakras and the organs and emotions that are associated with the chakra as an energy center within the body physically and energetically. Explain diamonds as amplifiers. Explain that the diamonds are amplifying the effects of the UV light.

Step 5: Let the client know that you will be providing visualization throughout the chakra work and up until the point that you begin the foot reflexology. Use a one of the visualizations provided or create your own.

Step 6: Instruct the client to get on the massage table in the supine position. Undergarments can be left on if it is comfortable for the client. It is appropriate to remove all other clothing.

Step 7: Open the session by placing a gem pillow down the center of the body and over the sheet that covers the client's body. Them gem pillow helps you to keep an eye on the gems, as they can get lost easily. The gem pillow should be made from all natural materials.

Step 8a: One by one begin placing the diamonds on the client.

Placement #1: root chakra: red light

Placement #2 sacral chakra: orange light

Placement #3 solar plexus: yellow light

Placement #4 heart chakra: pink/green light

Placement #5 throat chakra: blue light

Placement #6 third eye chakra: indigo/violet light

Placement #7 crowns chakra: white light

Step 8b: Describe each chakra and the ways that the particular influences of the stone will affect the chakra and the rest of the individual. Approx. 10 minutes.

Step 9: Perform inner smile visualization.

This is a Tao visualization… Imagine a place, person, or thing that you love very much. Hold the image in your mind until you can actually feel a smile come over your face. Try to hold that feeling of joy, love, and bliss. Now, turn that smile down towards yourself. Smile down on your own body and feel the love you felt towards your image, towards yourself now. Love every piece of you right now. Take a very thin golden blanket of light and cover your whole body with it. Take a big deep breath. As you move towards the feet from the crown chakra, do slow compressions down the client's body to bring focus and light to each part.

Step 10: Perform reflexology foot massage for 10-15 minutes.

Step 11: Finish with ankle balancing and compression from ankle to thigh.

Step 12: Sit at clients head and perform neck balancing and sacral compressions. Optional.

Step 13: Conclude session with your own manifestation for health. Thank the client through prayer for allowing you to work with them on this day. Look down on their body with love and compassion. Visualize a clean, balanced, and healthy human body lying in front of you. Remove diamonds from root to crown and thank the client verbally.

Soak diamonds in warm water with Sea salts to cleanse the stones properly. Remember to store the diamonds in a pouch made of natural fibers.

Protocol for diamond healing #2

1. Introduce the diamonds. Depending on the client's focus of healing, different colored stones and light will be used. Remember, colored light and colored diamonds are great for focus, but white light and stones can be used at all chakras. We want to determine from the beginning what area of focus the client wants to focus on: Spiritual balance, physical balance (injury/physical recuperation or stamina/energy/sexual balance), emotional balance, or mental balance.

2. Explain how focus will be brought to individuals through shiatsu pressure points, color light therapy, guided visualization, and diamond healing therapy at minor chakra points with a focus for balance within the seven major chakra centers.

3. Choose an appropriate aromatherapy oil based on the aspect of the persons being that the treatment is geared towards. Only natural/organic scents should be used. We use wood-based scents like cedar, pine, and sandalwood. We will use flower bases scents like lavender and rose. Herb based scents like rosemary and peppermint.

4. Tell the client that they should remove all of their clothing besides their underwear and to lie down on the bed face down and in between the covers.

    A heat lamp should be used to keep the client comfortable and to activate the molecular structure of the diamonds.

5. Let the client know that you are going to perform shiatsu therapy prior to the placement of each stone. The stones will be placed in this order:

    - One stone will be placed on the sole of each foot in the center following a shiatsu style massage.

    - One stone will be placed on the back of each knee following appropriate pressure points.

    - One stone will be placed at the root chakra

    - Practitioner will thumb up the 12 traditional bladder meridian points.

    - The practitioner will perform a head massage in the prone position and place a diamond at the 6th or 7th chakra to create a complete circuit of energy.

    ♋ One stone will be placed at each ear.

    ♋ Another set of stones will be placed on the inside of the cuneiform and in the center of each palm.

A total of 12 stones will be used during this treatment.

7.   Light therapy will begin at the soles of the feet, to the knee, and the sacral region. Special attention will be given to the chakra of interest and which that controls the balance the individual looks to create in his or her being. Each diamond will be charged with the light pen. One should hold the light pen as close as possible to the body. The practitioner should use their greater intuition when choosing which light to use where. The light pen should be used on each chakra for at least 1 minute-2 minutes.

8.   While charging the minor and major chakra points of focus the practitioner will be guiding the person through a visualization that focuses on peace and balance.

Example: Right now, we are focusing on the feet and nothing else. We are focusing on the weight they bear and we are going to take a conscious moment to recognize the responsibility we have in keeping them healthy and circulating. I would like you to feel the weight of your feet. I want you to see the light that I am using creating a prismatic burst of bright golden light slightly warming your feet and reminding you that they exist not separately from you, but as a part of you. I want you to hold the heat in your feet for a few moments and then slowly push it up your legs (all the while doing compressions from the achilles to anterior patella). I want you to notice how your legs feel. Do they feel heavy, do they hurt, do they tingle, and can you feel them at all? Remember the bright light that rests in your calves and push through the blockages you may feel here at your knees.

9.   Do a few circulating massage techniques pushing the physical energy in the legs up towards the heart. Follow with compressions up the legs to the sacrum and then up the bladder meridian to the head and then compress down each arm to the palm.

Example continued: Slowly feel the light moving from your feet to your knees to your lower back working its way through anything that may be blocking the flow on energy. Take as much time as you need to use this heat and light to scratch away at the physical and spiritual blocks that exist here at the sacrum. Move this energy and let it circulate slowly upwards to the top of your head. Now, feel your hands. How do they feel?

Do they feel heavy, tingly, sore, or do you feel nothing at all? Imagine a ball of light forming in the palms of your hands. First, imagine the light that I am using creating a circular path of light in your right palm and then slowly a flicker of light forms and with each pass over of the UV light pen, you see this flicker growing in size becoming larger and larger as if it is collecting and storing up the light. Imagine this happening until finally you are able to hold the image of a small ball of light in each hand. This light is your strength, your personal magnetism, and the will you have stored up until now in a hidden place in your body. With awareness, take each ball of light and shoot one up each arm. Send them up your arms beginning with the right one. Grab the light and will it up your arm to your elbow clearing physical blockages here and move it up to the back of the neck. Remembering now, that we have cleared the body up until the head; let the light rest in the region of your neck and cranial area. I want you to hold this vision for a few moments.

10. Sit at the head of the table and perform a head massage placing the stones appropriately.

   Ask your client to: take note of how they feel in their body.

11. Stand up, do a conscious chakra sweeping, and thank the client for their participation.

12. Remove the stones and exit the room.

Colors of stones: white, green, blue, brown, yellow, purple, pink, or red. All diamonds can be substituted for an alternative gemstone that is appropriate for the therapy.

Protocol for diamond healing #3

This treatment may be done using a diamond a pendulum

The treatment is meant to tune the energy of the body. This means that the circulatory system, the nervous system, and the endocrine system are all being subtly contacted and balanced. We will be using the C.D. called "Inside" by Paul Horn. We will be using aromas at the pulse points that correspond to the person's requested needs. We will begin by smudging the room or the client with sweet grass, cedar, or sage. It is not important that your client knows that you are clearing them, you may just burn a small amount under your table. The aroma reminds the person that something sacred is happening. The act of creating smoke actually changes the ionic structure in the air of the space and helps physically release any energy that has become attached to any subject. This energy then disperses in the air as the smoke carries it up and out. This gives the practitioner a more clean slate to work with.

The idea is that a chakra has a motion and a pulse just like any other organism that has been created by the great elements of the universe. Some atomic bonds are in rocks, some exist in water, and others exist is our blood, as well as most all things. One of the ways that we can determine if a chakra is out of balance is by using a pendulum. The practitioner holds the pendulum by its chain or string over the general area of the chakra being read. If the pendulum spins in an even spinning clockwise circle, it is in balance. The more oblong or askew the movement becomes, the more out of balance the chakra is. If the pendulum is still or moves in a counterclockwise motion, there is a block within the chakra and we will focus on bringing the energy back to this place by focusing on correcting the movement of the chakra through visualization and UV light therapy. You may use colored light or white light. Correspond colored light to the appropriate chakra color

Begin this treatment by giving a 10-minute foot massage to the client. Perform compressions up the body and arms. Perform a balancing neck massage for 5 minutes.

1st-7th chakra The treatment begins at the root chakra; using a pendulum to determine each particular chakras movement. Continue to read and balance the Chakras with the pendulum and the light pen.

If the chakra appears to be out of balance, use the light pen with the appropriate colored disc to balance the energy of the chakra. If the chakra is hardly leaking energy, use a high-energy color to raise the energy there. White, violet, and blue light all have the highest frequency of hertz vibrations. All light and diamond therapies should be accompanied by some sort of circulating massage to raise the blood flow and increase oxygen intake into all of the tissues in the physical body, preparing it to receive energy work. Singing bowls and tuning forks can add to this treatment as well.

You may end by having the client ask a question of the pendulum. Remind them that they are in one of the clearest places they've been for a while. Only perform this part if you feel comfortable doing it. Ask your client to ask questions with only yes or no answers. They will keep their eyes closed until the pendulum has a clear swing depicting the answer to their question. This brings the session to a close. Thank the client.

    If you have inquiries about obtaining any of the tools for healing listed in this book or you are interested in learning diamond therapy and obtaining more treatment protocols, please contact my web site at diamondtherapy.us

Bibliography

Bailey, Alice E.
> The Consciousness of an Atom
> Lucis Publishing Co. 1922-2000

Bloomfield, Louis A.
> How Things Work: The Physics of Everyday Life
> John Wiley & Sons, Inc. NY 1997

Brennan, Barbara Ann
> Hands of Light: A Guide to Healing through the Human Energy Field
> Bantam Press NewYork 1988

Capra, Fritjof
> The Tao of Physics
> A Bantum Book and Shambala Publications 1976

Carr-Gomm, Philip
> The Druid Tradition
> Element Press Rockport, Mass. 1995

Chia, Mantak and Maneewan
> Fusion of the Five Elements: Basic and Advanced Meditations for Transforming Negative
Emotions
> Healing Tao Books NY 1989

Devereux, Charla
> The Aromatherapy Kit
> Charles E. Tuttle Co. Boston 1993

Diagram Group, The
> The Facts on File Physics Handbook
> Diagram Visual Information Ltd. 2001

Foster, Steven
    The Book of the Vision Quest: Personal Transformation in the Wilderness
    A Fireside Book by Simon and Schuster NY 1992
Fritz, Sandy
    Fundamentals of Therapeutic Massage 2nd ed.
    Mosby Press, NY 2000
Hyemeyohsts Storm
    Seven Arrows
    Ballantine Books NY 1973
Jones, Wendy and Barry
    The Magic of Crystals: The Energy and Healing Power of Earth's Natural Wonders
    Harper & Collins Publishers 1996
Jordan, Michael
    Ceremonies for Life
    Collins & Brown Limited London 2001
Lee, William and Lynn
    The Book of Practical Aromatherapy
    Keats Publishing, Inc. New Canaan, Connecticut 1992
Lundberg, Paul
    The Book of Shiatsu
    A Fireside Book by Simon & Schuster Inc. N.Y. 1992
Matthews, John, and Various Author Contributions
    The World Atlas of Divination: The Systems: Where They Originate and How They
Work
    Headline Book Publishing 1994
McCoy, Edain
    Celtic Myth and Magik
    Llewellyn Publishing 1996

Page, R.I.

    Runes

    U of California Press/British Museum 1987

Patterson, Helena

    The Handbook of Celtic Astrology

    Llewellyn Publications 1995

Rattiseau, Elizabeth

    Magicians & Enchanters

    Laughing Elephant Seattle 2002

Swan, James A.

    Sacred Places: How the Living Earth Seeks Our Friendship

    Bear &Co.   Santa Fe NM 1990

Stover, Leon E. and Kraig, Bruce

    Stonehenge: The Indo-European Heritage

    Nelson Hall Chicago 1979

Wilks, William

    Science of a Witches Brew

    Maine Island Evergreen Estates, BC 1979

Weinstein, Marion

    Earth Magic: a Dianic book of shadows

    Phoenix Publishing WA. 1980

Ywahoo, Dhyani

    Voices of our Ancestors: Cherokee Teachings from the Wisdom Fire

    Shambhala Boston & London 1987

Magnolia May Polley

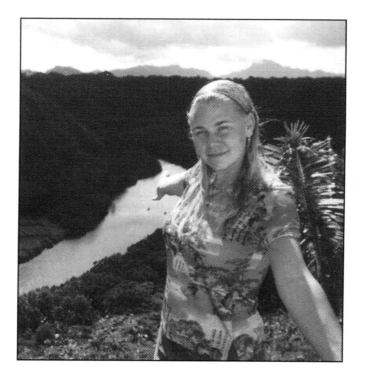

Wailua River, Kauai

Magnolia Polley currently works as the lead Massage Therapist for a premier spa in the Napa Valley. She has the spirit of an artist and a healer. Writing poetry and short stories since she was a child and able to pick up almost any type of art form with innate skill, she was naturally adept with her hands. Providing massage to her friends and family through her teenage years and always being influenced and interested in the mysteries of spirit and science, she was led to the field of the healing arts right out of high school. A native to the Pacific Northwest, Washington State is where she has spent most of her life. Magnolia's adventurous spirit has led her all over, but her heart still considers the small lake community of Chelan, nestled at the end of the Cascade Mountains, her home.

Printed in the United States
By Bookmasters